D1355655

Big is Invisible

Belinda Charlton

Big is Invisible

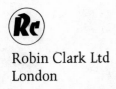

Robin Clark Ltd
London

First published by Robin Clark Limited 1985
A member of the Namara Group
27/29 Goodge Street, London W1P 1FD

British Library Cataloguing in Publication Data

Charlton, Belinda
  Big is invisible
  I. Reducing   II. Women — Health and hygiene
  I. Title
  613.2'5'0924   RM222.2

  ISBN 0-86072-087-X

Typeset by AKM Associates (UK) Ltd
Southall, Greater London
Printed and bound in Great Britain
by Mackays of Chatham Ltd, Kent

To Warwick, who loves me – through thick and thin

Contents

Big is Invisible

Introduction

I have been hungry all my life. As a baby, the youngest of three daughters, I was overfed by a doting mother. I was a bonny baby which, in my case, meant fat and lazy. When I was a teenager (11 stone) they called it puppy fat, but I was young and pretty and it did not bother me. As I grew older (12 stone) other euphemisms took over: cuddly, curvy, well-covered, pleasantly plump, chubby. Eventually, 'fat' became 'fat' and there followed a vicious circle of dieting, failing and comfort eating until I became gross (22 stone) and then very ill.

In the process I discovered that 'big' is invisible. When you grow as big as I did people make you feel you do not exist. I was ignored, as people ignore waiters. Eyes slid past me to focus on someone else. I was edited out of mind, made to feel part of the wallpaper. In response I tried to make myself unobtrusive, to withdraw into the sanctuary of anonymity.

Illness was the turning point. The prospect of ultimate invisibility *does* wonderfully concentrate the mind. In my instance it also kindled a fierce but irrational ambition, to transform myself, my body and my mind, and to compete in the London Marathon.

This meant that in two years I had to change from a 22-stone hulk who needed four nurses to lift her out of a hospital bed, to a 10-stone athlete, running joyfully over Westminster Bridge at the end of a 26-mile marathon.

The memory of that day will be with me for as long as I live.

The sun was shining, my body pouring with sweat, my muscles screaming with fatigue, but I was ecstatic.

The cheers of the crowd helped to lift me over the last few yards to the finish. Television reporters and photographers were on either side. At that moment I was probably the most visible woman in London, my image transmitted by television throughout the world. It was a spectacular ego trip. People were speaking of me as courageous and beautiful and an inspiration to others. My mail was equally flattering, invitations to be a guest of honour at luncheons and dinners, to give talks, open fêtes, judge competitions, make commercials and appear on television. Women implored me to help with their weight problems. Some men wrote to congratulate me, others wrote love letters.

My transformation from a 22-stone invalid to a marathon runner began when I lay in a hospital bed recovering from an operation for cancer of the uterus complicated by my vast weight. More than once I sensed my invisibility would be absolute. Although cancer was diagnosed I knew my weight was also the enemy. There was one moment when I felt I would welcome anything rather than put up with the pain and cold for a second longer. Then I realized what was happening: the pain and the freezing cold were proof I was still alive if rather short of blood. I heard a frightened voice inside me demand: 'Is this what you want with your life?' I appreciated, as I had never done before, that my life was the *real* thing. It was not a rehearsal or an action replay. This was it! I promised myself that if the pain and cold would go I would change. I promised to take life more seriously, to control myself and my appetites.

I was in intensive care following a five-hour operation. The pain did cease and the warmth of life did take over from the cold. For a year I went in and out of Southampton General Hospital for treatment. I vowed, if I survived, to be different. But survival was a longer, harder, more painful road than I could have imagined.

First, I had to understand properly how this had happened to me, to recognize my enemy – myself.

Part One

1 Getting There

I blamed my size on everything but eating. Low metabolism, genes, overactive/underactive glands, the cruel trick of a wicked fairy. I *did* have a low metabolism, a tendency to fat, but my weight was mostly due to gluttony, greed and delight in eating whenever, wherever and whatever I could.

Life offered me plenty of opportunities to indulge. At home my mother indulged me. When I became a young journalist my editors, through the generosity of expense accounts, indulged me. I married Warwick Charlton who travelled the world and took me with him to savour, sometimes with wonder, but always with approval, the best food the world could provide, prepared by some of the great chefs.

My husband had a bland, roast and two veg, taste acquired from his public school days and the Services. He regarded my great appetite, my acceptance of exotic foods, with admiring wonder. 'My wife is a gourmet,' he used to boast to friends, sometimes with real pride, but also, I suspected, to excuse my vast size. He used to beg me to diet, but I was cunning. I used delaying tactics and when the conversation got stuck on my size, skilfully changed the subject. My mother tried to persuade me to lose weight, she would have given anything in the world to have a beautiful slim daughter; she failed, her entreaties fell on a non-receptive mind.

I adored eating and my job as the show-business editor of

Trend, a magazine for girls, allowed me plenty of expense-account lunches, entertaining pop stars while interviewing them for my weekly 'profile' for the magazine. I ate and drank with them all: the Beatles, Rolling Stones and Kinks. I got fat – they got rich and famous.

While showing London how to swing in the sixties, I lived behind an Indian restaurant, the Curry Mahal on the Edgware Road, which was responsible for my addiction to curries.

It was at this time that I decided to try a trendy doctor's weight cure. He was a Harley Street consultant renowned for taking the flab off show-biz people. I was nearly 12 stone, not very overweight for me, but I wanted to look like Twiggy.

The doctor had his own, since discredited, method, quite acceptable to the relatively uninformed year of 1968. In fact his treatment was dangerous to the body and the mind: a three-month course of starvation (one apple a day) plus amphetamines, vitamins and unspecified daily injections. He made me strip naked to weigh in every day. For a poor weight loss the doctor gave me an admonitory slap on the bottom; a good weight loss earned an encouraging slap on the bottom. In the course of treatment I dropped from nearly 12 stone to 8, from an emotionally stable, hard working, hard-eating and drinking girl, to a well slapped, spaced-out pill popper.

Everybody said how beautiful I looked, but my brains were scrambled. It took time to recover from the 'cure'. During those three months of drugged starvation I was tormented by the delicious aromas from the Curry Mahal. I could not escape the fragrant smell of curry when in my flat. It became an obsession. As soon as I went off the doctor's diet, I promised myself, I would treat myself to a curry.

I did not let myself down. I went into the Curry Mahal for a celebratory vindaloo, and then kept on going back. I did not finally emerge from curry restaurants for ten years.

I loved all foods but especially exotic food. I also put on pounds eating everyday food. I ate bigger helpings of everything and then, when no one was watching, the best of the leftovers. Even after a meal at one of the best gourmet restaurants in the world I would go back to the hotel for a light snack, an omelette or club sandwich before bed.

A lot of this could be classified as comfort eating, but I also enjoyed the taste, texture, smell and colour of the food. In Thailand I ate snake, in Egypt I ate camel and chocolate-covered bumble-bees from Fortnum and Mason.

My most memorable curry was in Sri Lanka, and was served on the terrace of the Galle Face Hotel, Colombo. The orchestra played a selection of Ivor Novello melodies in the background. Waiters padded soft-footed to and from our table. A large fan stirred the velvet night air and the lights from the cruise liners, anchored offshore, shone in the Indian Ocean. It was all so redolent of the Raj; I half expected to see Somerset Maugham entertaining Noel Coward and Dickie Mountbatten at the next table. The curry was pungently aromatic to my taste and served with dozens of dainty side dishes.

I enjoyed eating so much, that I didn't see the signs that it was seriously affecting my life. I was leading such a busy life bringing up three of my seven stepchildren, that I ignored the fact that my weight was going up and up.

Almost without realizing it, I had reached the point of no return. It was no longer a case of being pleasantly plump. I was vast . . . horrendous. I had gone well over what was acceptable. I really looked obscene – and I weighed well over 20 stone. At my heaviest I must have weighed at least 22 stone and at that size you don't really notice if your weight has gone up a stone or two! In any case I was too big to weigh myself on the scales.

Eventually people stopped teasing me about my weight because it just wasn't funny any more. It was embarrassing instead – for them and me.

I tried to pretend the problem did not exist by refusing to look at myself in the mirror. I tried to fool myself that I hadn't really changed underneath. I had, of course. There were all sorts of things that I couldn't do because of my weight. I couldn't carry a box of groceries because my stomach got in the way. I couldn't get in the back of a Mini or fasten my seat belt in a plane. I couldn't hug or cuddle my stepchildren. I couldn't even have my hair done – the gown wouldn't go on and I couldn't fit in the chair.

Not only could I not fit into chairs, I used to break them. At a dinner party my hosts would often send for an especially sturdy chair as they thought, quite rightly, that a normal chair might not be strong enough.

Between us my husband and I broke beds in hotels around the world. He is 6ft 3 inches and also overweight, so the two of us represented a serious challenge to hotel furniture.

In a hotel on Sunset Boulevard in Los Angeles we set a record by breaking two beds in one night. My bed broke, all four legs gave way with a terrifying thud, so I crawled into my husband's bed and broke that as well. The guests in the room below ours must have wondered what was happening!

As I grew bigger people became more distant. In Ringwood, our local market town, they rarely stopped to chat in shops or the street as they do now. They used to remember my name (I was very recognizable) but would rarely pass the time of day. This was mostly due to my lack of confidence which made me surly and withdrawn; in any case I was probably hurrying to my next meal!

The addiction to food is harder to give up than anything else. We can all give up drinking and smoking, sometimes forgetting the pleasures they may have given in the past. Food will not let go of you so completely, you can never give it up entirely. Most failed dieters will agree that it is easier to eat almost nothing for a week, than to eat three moderate meals a day. Therefore it is not enough just to diet, we fatties have to battle for the rest of our lives with the obese person trying to take over the slim one.

I knew it would take drastic action to fight the glutton in me, or at least to arrange a compatible truce.

As an invisible person no one ever asked my advice but I had plenty to give. I knew more about dieting and the secret excesses of a foodaholic than anyone. I'd made up more excuses for my size than a room full of fatties at a slimming club. I'd hidden more bars of chocolate under the bed, eaten more leftovers standing by the kitchen sink, than I care to remember. On one occasion I stood at the open fridge and ate a plateful of cold spaghetti with my fingers. Yes, I knew all about the secret vices of a food addict.

But part of getting fat was also fun: the mouth-watering sorbet at the Madison in Washington DC; the pork and apricot dish at Butterfields on Sunset Boulevard; the classically simple steak with the not so simple Bernaise sauce at the Petit Zinc in Paris; fresh sardines served alfresco in a grubby cafe in Estoril crisped over an open fire; fragrant crunchy chips and creamy fresh cod from the Sea Shell Chippie in Lisson Grove, London; enchilladas with 'sock-it-to-me' Margueritas at La Fonda, Ensinada, Mexico; solidly sensible scrumptious steak-and-kidney pie at the Wig and Pen in the Strand; delicious steak-and-kidney pudding, oozing rich gravy at the French Horn, Sonning.

North Chinese, Thai and Indian cooking are my favourite foods. I do not know how many stones of extra weight they represented of my 22 stone, but I do know that, in China, I remember the Great Wall far less vividly than I do the Peking Duck in Peking, which was served with wafer-thin pancakes, rich plum sauce and crunchy vegetables. Another more humble dish, difficult to identify but which I call Dragon Chow Mein, had the most delicate and subtle flavours I can remember.

I needed little encouragement to eat anywhere, but a good atmosphere was enough to stimulate my excesses. In the United States, for example, at a smart riverfront seafood restaurant in Boston, I ate lobster, crayfish, oysters and clam in such quantities and with such slurping abandon that it resembled nothing so

9

much as the erotic eating scene from the movie *Tom Jones*. The impressed manager announced he planned to rope off the table and mark it with a plaque 'Belinda ate here – X rated'.

My favourite eating place of all is not in the United States (although for overall high standard America would certainly rival Paris) but in England. It is the Mallory Court Hotel near Leamington Spa. The atmosphere is that of a magnificently run English country house, the menu is small but exquisite, the Grand Marnier soufflé is perfection and would tempt me now ... It was all very well for me to recall my culinary delights, laugh at the work I put in with my knife and fork, chopsticks and even fingers, but there was a price to pay and only part of it could be satisfied with credit cards.

The pounds settled remorselessly upon me. Despite my diets and guilt-ridden visits to health farms, I got bigger, moved more slowly and thought hardly at all. I became less effective in almost everything I did. I convinced myself that I enjoyed my life, but it wasn't true any longer. It was on my thirty-third birthday when some young relatives decided to give me a treat, that I realized how far I had slipped.

They did up my hair, made up my face, dug out one of my 'tent' dresses from the back of my wardrobe and presented me to the waiting guests in the dining room. Presents were laid out on the table with a birthday cake (small so as not to tempt me). Someone said how nice I looked with my hair in little plaits; I caught sight of my smiling fat face in the mirror. I was thirty-three years old, I looked at least forty-five, and I was being treated like an old lady. My hosts agreed in whispers (assuming that I was not only fat, but half-witted and deaf) that I should be encouraged to do something about my eating, that *it was bad for my health*. It was well meant, I suppose, but I didn't really appreciate it. I had so little energy. I had long known that my ability to cope with the daily business of living was slowing down.

Then came a period when my greatest achievement of the day

was getting up and dressed and into the car. Even that was an alarming ordeal. After a short drive I was exhausted. I swore I would curb my appetite, but inevitably betrayed myself.

Not long after my thirty-third birthday my gradual decline reached an all-time low. Cancer was diagnosed. My husband was deeply shocked. I accepted the news with a mixture of horror and relief. At least, I told myself, this was not my fault, and I did not have to struggle along on my own, blaming my own undoubted inadequacies. Now doctors, nurses and medical science had to take over.

But even when the mental agony of the radium treatment, the operation and convalescence was over, I knew (in the dark cave of my mind) that a fearful problem remained. The surgeon's knife had neither removed nor tempered my appetite, my insatiable craving for food. There was a solution to my problem and it came from an unexpected source. At the time it seemed pure folly prompted by desperate optimism.

2 Next to Last Enemy

It was a tremendous relief to be free of the burden of guilt I had carried so long. For once, this was something not 'my fault'. There was little I could do, it was up to the doctors who assured me that cancer of the uterus was curable if it could be diagnosed in the early stages as mine had been. Of course, they were not sure until they opened me up, so I lay back and resigned myself to the treatment. I was in and out of hospital for nearly a year for tests or radiotherapy. There was a nightmarish week when I was packed full of radium and shut in a room on my own. I had to lie in my back and try to keep still for six days. Food was pushed at me three times a day, but because of the risk of radiation exposure nursing was minimal. It was very unpleasant but there was nothing I could do. I felt my family was probably suffering far more than I was, particularly my husband and my mother.

Although I was frightened by my illness, and vowed to have a greater respect for my life when I came out of hospital, I did not go on a diet straight away. I did not really accept that my recovery was placed in jeopardy by my weight. Other women in hospital with me for similar operations were back at work in two months and living normally. I found it difficult to plan a normal day: housework, a trip to the shops, preparing some meals, typing a few letters. By midday I was shattered.

I discovered I could get a little surge of energy with a couple of stiff vodkas. Because I was ill and nothing was my fault, I indulged myself. I ate anything I fancied and drank what I liked. My days became bolstered with vodka, my evenings a semi-conscious haze. My energy level was at an all-time low and I found concentration hard. Reading was an impossibility: I could not take in a whole television programme. My illness and the radiation treatment had left me with the side effect of a massive depression.

In hospital I had lost 3 stone in weight, but only three months later I was getting fatter and on my way back to the 22-stone mark. People reassured me, my life was saved, I was cured and had a wonderful future. My depressed self told me that I was miserable, incompetent, prematurely middle aged. I would never enjoy travelling the world with my husband again, enjoy dancing, swimming or walking. I longed for some physical activity, but never felt fit enough. I longed for the possibility (not necessarily the reality) of another man in my life to prove I was as attractive as I used to be. But who would want me?

I promised everyone I would diet, but every failure made me even more depressed. During my life of dieting I had tried every method of losing weight – and failed with them all.

There was the Hollywood powdered protein diet which actually came with a money-back guarantee, but you had to be a millionaire to sue and it had me guzzling gallons of the hellbrew to no effect. There was the Formula 21 diet which had me swallowing a substance that worked like cotton wool, the stuff swelled in your stomach to make you feel full. I did not feel full, just pregnant and hungry. I tried the grapefruit diet which put me off grapefruit for life.

The Beverley Hills diet made me unpopular at other people's homes and restaurants when I turned up with my own supply of pineapples. The 'F' plan diet had me munching a nosebag like a horse full of oats and bran. I tried the high protein diet, but that got too expensive, and if I saw another salad again I swore I would scream. I gave up counting calories because my maths was too shaky.

I tried the substitute diets – the 'meal in a biscuit' – which spoiled my appetite for a proper meal. I never ate anything *instead* of something else only *as well as*. I did learn, though, from my diets, that the best aid to food appreciation is a really good appetite. Very often overweight people never allow themselves to get very hungry. I discovered that really to enjoy food, you need to be extremely hungry. No culinary credits or exotic sauces can be a substitute for starvation as a real gourmet experience. That is why food appreciation and bingeing are two separate things – one aesthetic, the other emotional.

I was a gourmandizing binger. If I knew I had something really good to eat, I used to conserve my appetite, eating nothing. After a meal I deemed it safe to binge. A dreadful combination.

Meanwhile my visits to the hospital for cancer checks lengthened from monthly to three monthly. If all went well, they assured me, it would be only twice a year, and then an annual checkup.

Medical science had given me a new life, but I did not think I had much use for it. Three months out of hospital, despite the good resolutions, my ability to battle had disappeared.

I saw visitors to my home as adversaries, representing extra meals to be cooked, beds changed and problems to sort out. Concentration became so difficult I sometimes picked a quarrel with Warwick, my husband, so he would not speak to me.

Of course I knew people were hurt and puzzled by my behaviour, but I could do nothing! My life was totally self-engrossed, I had no room for anyone else.

All the time I planned my next move. Each action was rehearsed in my mind a dozen times: picking up a coffee cup, walking to the kitchen, turning on the cooker, preparing the vegetables. Having done that I would sit down and rest while preparing my next move, until finally I had cooked and dished up a meal. The effort of talking to anyone at the meal table dismayed me. I sat there in stunned exhaustion, then ran off, shut myself in the bedroom or bathroom to prepare for the next stage of washing the dishes. I am sure there would have been plenty of willing helpers in my family, but I reasoned that, if I did any less, I would make myself redundant and be even more depressed. There seemed no escape. I was willing to try anything.

3 Like a Bird

One afternoon I sat, a tin of biscuits and a bottle of pop beside my chair, in front of the television, watching the London Marathon. More than anything I envied the competitors the energy and self-discipline necessary to run over 26 miles. The people on my screen were not super-athletes, but ordinary people running for fun, for a sport; for the dedicated few it was a way of life. I had never run, or done anything athletic, but used to love walking in the forest. The running I watched on television seemed an escape, a freedom, like a kite or a bird soaring.

My stepson Randal was running in that marathon, and he and I were much the same age. When he came down the following weekend to the Gothic castle where I lived, I told him I thought the marathon a marvellous achievement.

He said that it had changed his whole attitude to life: made him calmer, more able to cope with stress, to cut down on drinking and lose weight; altogether, made him a happier and more contented person. Randal told me that running had a plus, a secret bonus. And what was that? Ah, he mumbled mysteriously, I would have to find out for myself.

'Why don't you have a go?' he said. 'I will be your trainer.'

The idea seemed preposterous. I could barely heave myself out of my armchair, let alone run any distance and certainly not 26 miles.

But the seed was sown. I bought some books on running and

discovered it was advocated as a cure for depression by some doctors.

I also read a tantalizing item: that noradrenalin, released through running into the bloodstream, gave a lift, a feeling of happiness, a surge of euphoric well-being. In his book, *The Complete Jogger*, Bruce Tulloh confirmed the runner's 'high' as a 'pretty good' feeling. The *Three As* manual also suggested running would give you a buzz. A medical journal said women often benefited from running during the change of life because it helped sort out hormonal problems and lifted depression.

But nowhere did I find anything that recommended the advisability of jogging for a 22-stone woman, particularly one recovering from a major illness. I did read though that anyone more than 15 pounds overweight should consult a doctor before jogging. I doubted if a doctor would consider me suitable jogging material; nevertheless, the idea had taken root.

Randal's first training instructions arrived by post on 13 May 1982. My new life had begun.

'All sorts of shapes and sizes were running in the Marathon,' he wrote. 'Women with conference-pear bums, men with Heineken-lager bellies, geriatrics with paramedic assistants, comedians with emus and horses' heads, as well as the slim fit ones.'

This was encouraging for a start. Then followed the week's training instructions:

Sunday	Go for a walk. Time it and report.
Monday	Walk five minutes briskly.
Tuesday	Walk five minutes slowly.
Wednesday	Walk ten minutes slowly.
Thursday	Walk fifteen minutes (stop and rest if you want).
Friday	Rest.
Saturday	Walk five minutes.

'Drink as much as you like [goodie!] but do not exceed more

than one bottle of vodka a day; drink as much wine as you like. Do not attempt suicide. Eat as much as you like.'

This looked like a doddle. There was no talk of running, so no possible warning from a doctor about the dangers of overdoing it.

I was in a pit of depression. Running was an escape route. Reading about that runner's high was also intriguing; by all accounts it was usually achieved on a long run. I also brightened to learn that runners had to eat lots of carbohydrates two or three days before a long run; pasta, biscuits, chocolate, bread and potatoes all figured in a marathon runner's diet which cheered me up no end. Talking to runners tempered my optimism. Ahead were months of sustained effort, hunger, sore joints, aching limbs, breathlessness, blistered feet and physical pain. There were also rewards: the feeling of achievement, pride, self-satisfaction and a new self-respect, a driving force to take me through the hard training months to the ultimate goal of the London Marathon.

For my first day of training I dressed carefully with a sense of occasion, wore my favourite dress, an overcoat, stout brogue shoes and carried a handbag. All set to go, I made one mistake and forgot to lock up our Birman cat, Theo, who followed me. The first few yards he stayed undercover until I was too far from home to turn back, then he hopped out on to the road to surprise me. So instead of a brisk and purposeful training walk I had to scramble through the rhododendron bushes, other people's gardens and over fences to try to catch Theo.

We arrived home together, Theo in my arms, swearing, and me covered in mud and scratches, but I was stimulated by the excitement and exercise. For the first time for two years I did not feel depressed and in need of a large vodka or slice of chocolate cake. I felt pleased, hopeful that my new regime would continue to make me feel better, although, of course, I would probably never run a marathon – but it was a harmless aspiration.

I recorded in my diary the distance covered each day, and the time it took. My first piece of running equipment was not a pair of shoes or a tracksuit, but a stop-watch. After each training walk I recorded distance and time and developed a code. A typical diary entry was as follows:

W. 30 mins, I ml. Felt awful B & F.

This meant that I had walked for thirty minutes and covered one mile, felt awful and had been drinking and smoking the previous day (hence B & F – booze and fags).

Monday:	W. 10 mins. Felt awful B & F.
Tuesday:	W. 20 mins (little better, no B & F).
Wednesday:	Nothing.
Thursday:	W. 30 mins (very windy had to stop).
Friday:	Rest.
Saturday:	W. 10 mins. Felt awful WD (withdrawal symptoms, i.e., hangover).

This predictably confirmed the harmful effects of drinking and smoking, but I also discovered running was a cure, the only one, for a hangover. A 5-mile run cleared a merry evening's indulgence, a three-bottles-of-wine job took twice the distance.

Gradually, my walks got longer as I explored the New Forest. In just two weeks I was walking faster without getting short of breath. I remembered how I used to set out on walks ten minutes before the rest of the family because of the hill outside the castle, where we lived. I used to have to rest halfway up the hill and then stop to catch my breath at the top. It was always an embarrassment trying to keep up. Now, I soon found I could walk up the hill without a break for a rest.

Another reward was a new awareness of all the sights and sounds around me. I heard the noises made by the wind in the trees, the silver birch light and bustling like the rustle of a crisp cotton petticoat; the whooshing sound of the oak; and as the rhododendrons bloomed my walks were heavily perfumed.

Soon I grew more adventurous. My husband Warwick joined me, but it was not all brightness and light despite the undoubted coming-alive feeling. One six-mile walk in the Forest got us lost and cross; we ended up walking 15 miles and not speaking to each other.

A good part of the walk was over wet and marshy heathlands, through woods, over banks of squelchy mud and streams. Warwick pulled me over into a particularly ripe and smelly bog, so I hurried ahead and let him traverse a wet marshland unaided while I watched his struggles, out of sight by the roadside. He was lost, his anguished bellows left me unmoved, but not the unfortunate picnickers who had settled by the roadside. The sound of Warwick's roars halted their feast. For a moment the family froze, then Mum, Dad, Gran and assorted kids hurriedly packed the sausage rolls, scotch eggs and individual fruit pies back into the basket with scared glances in the direction of the wood and Warwick's cries of anguish; they scurried into their car and made off.

Warwick soon emerged still roaring his frustration and very wet. I calmed him with a large cream tea: scones, strawberry jam and cakes in the New Forest Tea Room in Burley.

The pitfalls of the New Forest were not only bogs and marsh-land. I had been making earnest efforts to eat sensibly, not really dieting, but not bingeing or over-eating. Forest walks seemed fine, I would not be tempted to eat trees or leaves – but I had not allowed for the cream-tea factor. There is nowhere in the New Forest too remote to harbour a tea room or hotel which serves delicious cream teas. Along with curry, cream teas are my other secret vice. Indeed, Warwick and I spent our honeymoon flitting from cream tea to cream tea, like particularly massive butterflies.

The cream-tea factor in the Forest was likely to be my undoing. It was a relief, therefore, that four weeks after I started the training walks, I was ready to try my first run.

4 First Run

I wore a smart dress and coat, walking shoes and carried my handbag. I wanted to be sure that if anybody saw me they would think I was running for a bus or chasing a dog. I set my stop-watch and ran along the old railway line for as long as I could, until my heart was pounding, my bosom heaving, my legs like jelly and my breath came in rasping gasps. I thought I had run for at least ten minutes and covered half a mile. The stop-watch told a different story:

Time run thirty seconds. Distance covered about 100 metres.

My second run was not much better. It was in the New Forest with Warwick.

Diary

2 June 1982

We struck right into the heart of the Forest today. It was dark and dense with only the birds, witches and goblins to witness our efforts. We ploughed further into the woods, feeling the heavy presence of 600-year-old oaks. On the air hung a sweet sickly scent, rather like candy floss. Small creatures scurried as we approached and a deer flitted nervously in the distance. Then out of the heart of the dark forest, something stirred. Around an oak tree appeared a pair of red running shorts attached to a sweating jogger. Was nothing sacred? He ignored us, and the awesome dignity of the oaks, and crashed through the forest, his mind obviously set on 'personal bests'.

Spurred on by his example, I decided to have another go myself. This would be the first time Warwick had seen me run.

I ran for about half a minute, and stopped completely exhausted. When Warwick stopped laughing he told me I looked like a badly upholstered camel, humps swaying from side to side. I invited him to have a go, to see if he could do better, but he declined.

Soon I was running for a few more seconds every day. It was agony. It then occurred to me to make things a little easier for myself. One day I went out without my handbag. It felt like letting go of the rail of a swimming pool. I was on my own. I was a jogger, no longer pretending to catch a bus or exercise the dog. The time had come to buy a tracksuit and the rest of the runner's gear.

In the sports shop in Ringwood I said I was shopping for my son Michael who was big, about my size. Then my husband came bounding into the shop and announced proudly that I had taken up jogging, and would they fit me out? I hid in the changing cubicle feeling foolish, but there was no escape, so I squeezed and hauled my 22-stone body into the biggest tracksuit in the shop. It was as tight as a sausage skin, but comfortable, and I grew to love it dearly. Then came the shoes, Nike Pegasus, especially well cushioned in the heels to protect from jarring (they would be taking my full weight at each step). Socks were also important, thick and unseamed to cushion the feet, protect from blisters and absorb perspiration, and large enough not to cramp the feet; again I chose Nike.

I loved my new tracksuit and shoes – symbols of hope. Each night I folded them up carefully and put them on the chair. The shoes went on a small bedside table at the end of the bed where I could see them. In the morning I went through a routine: first of all, on with my track suit, shoes laced carefully and tied neatly. I put on my stop-watch, smeared vaseline on my face to prevent wind soreness, and tied a blue headband around my hair.

The slow walk down the stairs of the Castle and out of the front door seemed an eternity. I would dread what lay before me but was quite unable to turn back. I never cut short my training programme, to do so would have been a confession of failure and I could not cope with that. I had enough trouble controlling my eating and drinking. Usually I was followed by my cat, Theo. Together we faced the grim, often cold early morning. Theo quivered with excitement and anticipation at the promise of the day, while I felt sick with apprehension at the physical and mental struggle ahead.

The morning looked beautiful, mist swirling lazily off the River Avon snaking along the edge of the Castle grounds. I watched the cows drinking at the water's edge as the tangerine sun rose above the trees. The geese and swans seemed oblivious of onlookers, and sometimes a family of deer would be startled by my presence.

My first aim, when I began to run, was to cover non-stop a quarter of a mile of a 1-mile circuit. This took me to the white-post landmark in our drive, and I still shudder at the memory of the effort of those early painful days when running to the white post seemed to be stretching myself on a torturer's rack. My diary for one of those days is a reminder:

Diary

Every time I run it hurts. I cannot believe I am really inflicting this pain on myself every day. Every inch of the way is agony. I count my breaths and I count the driveways along the road. I wait for the landmarks like the white post at the halfway mark, a pretty thatched cottage at the top of a small hill. I know I'll feel a bit better over the hill. Then follows a long straight bit. I desperately want to stop now. All I have to do is stand still, but I never do. I always carry on. To give up would be to admit defeat, and I will not be defeated.

Thump, thump . . . I listen to the rhythm of my feet hitting the tarmac drive. I look at the trees and marvel at the outline of the leaves against the sky. I smell different scents and try to distinguish them, but most of all I listen to myself breathing. I tell myself that if I breathe rhythmically I can make it to the end of the drive, make it to one gatepost and then I'll make it to the next. All I have got to do is make it to the letter box. Past the letter box and then I'll know I can make it to the end of the drive once again. The feeling afterwards is terrific. Walking back home is wonderful. I have run half a mile and am on top of the world.

The devils and gremlins which jostle my brain when I first wake up have been banished for another twenty-four hours. Checking the time on my watch is exciting. Maybe I will have knocked a few seconds off my previous 'best time'.

I was beginning to learn some runner's jargon. A 'PB' is a Personal Best and the highlight of every run was to see if I had shaved off a second or two.

I used to talk intensely to anyone who would listen about my 'times', the inclines in the road, 'hillwork' and 'interval running', discuss the relative merits of different road surfaces, tarmac versus grass, cobbles versus ploughed fields. I was in danger of becoming, like a lot of joggers, rather too committed to the cause and failing to see the funny side to the sport.

The joggers who gave up drinking and went on a strict diet three months before a competitive run, were probably doing the right thing by the book, but I thought them too obsessed. They made me aware that the running could take over, the cure could become the sickness. I was determined to keep it in perspective. It was a great relaxer and tension reliever, a miracle cure for a hangover, it did put sparks in the bedroom, restore self-respect and was a healthy substitute for valium. Running allowed me to speak with confidence and composure to bank managers, traffic wardens or the police officer delivering a summons.

If I could not go for a run I became agitated. I would later run myself to a state of exhaustion and then fall asleep. I met one man who claimed to run a marathon every weekend. I took a vow that I would not say, as he did more than once a day, 'Running has changed my life'. I would not let slip to everyone that I managed to 'do' a couple of miles every morning, and then try to look appropriately modest. I would not treat fellow runners as 'soul mates' belonging to a secret society on a higher level to mortal folk. I promised myself that I would not talk continuously about 'personal bests' or 'cramps' or 'runner's nausea' or 'sore knees'. I vowed not to talk about 'the wall' at all. I would not read more than one book about running a week or be incredibly abrupt to the telephone caller who was holding up my run.

Most of all I promised that I would not secretly hug myself with self-satisfaction and feel superior to all non-runners. I would keep my running enthusiasm within bounds although, without my early morning run, even on dark wet mornings, I would feel uncomfortable and twitchy like a junkie without a fix.

I was obviously hooked but, listening to experienced runners, I heard there really was a 'fix', a 'runner's high', but it was to be many, many miles of running before I found that elusive 'fix' for myself.

5 Caroline Bakes a Cake

Running made me feel good enough to start to diet seriously and to join the local Weight Watchers' slimming club in Ringwood to help speed up my weight loss.

My husband came along for moral support. I weighed 18 stone 10 pounds and was easily the fattest person present. I paid my subscription, filled in a form and skulked as usual, like most very fat people, in an inconspicuous corner of the room.

I was given a goal weight of 10 stone 3 pounds, an 8 stone 8 pounds weight loss in addition to the three stone plus I had already lost through running. My diary shows how I felt.

Diary

13 July 1982

Walked back from Ringwood today 2½ miles with heavy shopping in a rucksack on my back. Hated the extra weight, cursed it all the way back. Vowed I wouldn't carry shopping again when walking. When I got home I weighed the shopping. It was 21 pounds, less than half the amount of weight I have already lost. How on earth will I feel in the unlikely event of my losing 119 pounds?

Back at Weight Watchers I noticed that many of the women

looked bright and smart as though they did not need to lose anything. These were women who were close to their goal weight or else had reached their goal and were on maintenance. The slimming club told me to weigh everything I ate and to eat only what was written in the programme they gave me.

This was mostly fish and chicken, with salads and green vegetables. I was allowed meat three times a week, the occasional ice cream or digestive biscuit, three slices of bread a day or three small potatoes. The diet was very varied and sensible but, nevertheless, I found it quite difficult to keep to. The dieting programme insisted on moderation, and moderation was not something I was very good at. I decided to work out my own diet. But getting weighed by an independent person is a good discipline.

I believe it is easier to eat very little, so as not to stimulate your appetite or taste buds, than to eat three moderate meals a day. I often would eat only one, a generous evening meal. This method is frowned upon by some experts who maintain that what you eat at night takes longer to digest and the calories are not burned up in bed. But I managed better on one good meal at night. It helped me to sleep and cut down the time I was involved with eating to once a day. I certainly lost weight my way.

Eating very little during the day also fitted in well with those early days of running.

After a difficult run the last thing you want to do is eat. But you do need to drink and I drank dozens of cups of decaffeinated coffee with skimmed milk and artificial sweetener.

At lunch time I was still tired from my run and was satisfied with a little fruit or natural yoghurt.

By the early evening I was usually really hungry and ate a fairly normal main meal, but made an effort to cut out red meat, animal fats, refined sugar and all sweets, puddings, cakes, biscuits and thick sauces.

I zoomed in on Low Cal. Anything marked Low Cal I went for,

the orange juice, fizzy drinks, soups, frozen foods, salad creams. The truth, of course, is that water is the best low cal drink, or nothing at all.

It is difficult to stick to any diet, especially if you are worried. A calm, peaceful, controlled frame of mind is the most important part of losing weight and I got that from running.

In one of the many anguished days when I fell off the waggon I wrote in my Diary.

Diary

Sneaked off and had a big stinky curry, followed by two packets of shortbread biscuits and ice cream. Went to bed with a box of chocolates. Felt dreadful.

I broke my regime many times, sometimes with surprising results. On one occasion I had succumbed to some wine after a poor run in the morning.

Diary

30 August 1982

For the first time I am unable to complete 6/10 of a mile or even 3/10. My morning run was delayed and the afternoon excursion to the fair loomed up. Climbed into the car with Warwick and the children and drove to the top of the drive. I remember the instructions of Randal, my trainer, who said that absolutely nothing must come in the way of my daily run. I decided to postpone it no longer. To the surprise of Warwick and the children, I parked the car and announced I would go for a run before the outing to the fair.

To my horror, after struggling for a few yards, I was

exhausted and had to stop. I tried again but managed only 200 yards. My legs were wobbling and breath terribly laboured. I walked and staggered and ran for 4/10 of a mile and then gave up. I slunk back to the car to Warwick and the children, feeling disgusted with myself.

That evening I was really fed up and had a few glasses of wine. Then a few more. Finally I decided to stop all the nonsense and go out once more and do a proper run. By this time I had drunk quite enough Dutch Courage, nearly two bottles of wine.

It was magic. I ran effortlessly in the dark with none of the usual landmarks to worry me and none of the pain. I felt I was flying, and without the customary quarter and halfway marks because of the darkness, felt freed of all restrictions. I was running just for the joy of being alive. For the first time ever, I was disappointed when I saw the posts at the end of the drive which signalled the end of the run. When I arrived home I was on a special high – I had no hangover or indeed any desire to drink more. Just wonderfully exhilarated. The family who had been forced to feed themselves during my absence, were not upset or critical of my slight inebriation. They seemed to share some of my euphoria. My stepdaughter Caroline had even baked a cake.

6 Dieting Tricks

The dieting was, and is, and always will be, the hardest part of all. It is in my nature that, if a little of something tastes good, then a whole lot more tastes a whole lot better. Enough is not as good as a feast, a feast is much better.

If I was to have any hope of success I knew I had to analyse my behaviour: discover when I ate so much and how to prevent the habit.

First, I established that a sensible meal, instead of satisfying hunger, merely stimulated my appetite for more.

Putting off eating as late into the day as possible worked for me. Getting out of the habit of eating several times a day was also a good discipline. The first day was hell, but I knew it could not last forever, the second day was a bit easier, and on the third day I had begun to find non-eating activities to replace breakfast and lunch. I did at last find the trick – do nothing to encourage the demon appetite.

By cutting out fattening foods for as long as possible, I sometimes lost the taste for them. This was certainly the case with red meats, fats and strong flavourings, even curry, so often the cause of my previous downfalls.

To escape from eating situations I used to go to the woods or the garden, work out in the gymnasium or do some aerobics. If I could not get out of the house, I used to set up the ironing board in a part of the house furthest from the kitchen, perhaps in the spare bedroom or the bathroom, then iron furiously for as long as it took to get over my craving for food, usually between twenty minutes and two hours. I used to save up the ironing just for this sort of emergency.

Sitting in the sauna or having a sunbed was another way to escape eating. Sometimes I used to have tape cassettes on all the time, buy a new cassette at lunchtime instead of eating and spin out the business of choice. I made a visit to an art gallery or a country house, or a new hobby like embroidering a tablecloth or painting a picture, a substitute for eating: anything to occupy hands that could otherwise be popping food into my mouth.

I used to think of all the non-eating things I liked to do and make lists. I established the different places not associated with food, like churches or hardware stores. I tried not to eat on buses or in the car or out on the street while shopping, to limit all food-associated activities. Food shopping was strictly once a week. The family suffered because I would not buy anything that might tempt me.

When I was in a car I trained myself to look at non-food-associated places, to skip restaurants and food stores, and count banks, insurance offices, travel agents, car showrooms, estate agents and clothes shops.

Diary

Short walk, swim 10 lengths.

Very hungry so decided to forget about eating with a visit to the new Sport Recreation Centre in Ringwood with Warwick, Alex and Eileen (stepson and wife). It is very grand with a big pool, squash courts, massage and beauty-treatment rooms obviously built with a pre-Thatcher budget. It was very bright and bold on the lines of the Pompidou Exhibition Centre in

Paris where they show brightly painted pipes and everything is designed as though with a child's building blocks, and a great deal of glass. It raised Hampshire eyebrows when it was built, but I think it is magnificent and has everything (including queues of people).

Then I went to the beauty-treatment area which is called the Roman Rooms, small but bright and attractive with very friendly attendants. Here they stroke and pummell and caress you. When it first opened a few dirty old men hovered hopefully outside hoping to catch a glimpse of naked nubile lasses; all they actually see are naked dirty old men, and me, swathed in an enormous pink towel looking like a moist pink blancmange. The solarium is like a space capsule. It takes me twenty minutes to wedge my bulk between the two grills of ultra-violet light. It gets extremely hot and I wondered if I would be shot out of the machine when I was done. When the heat gets to screaming point it turns itself off; by this time you are lying in a pool of water and so begin the wriggling sliding gymnastics which are needed, for someone of my bulk, to get out of the machine. Stark naked and lying half in the machine and half on the floor, you pray no one comes in. Like a sea-lion emerging from the water, you make one more gigantic wriggle and land on the floor with a plop, hot, wet and beached. Next my eyebrows were plucked for the first time. It is marginally better than the dentist but there is not much in it.

Then I went for a shower and was slightly surprised to see a naked man, very slowly showering next to me. He seemed a little disappointed that it was me, but decided bravely to make the best of it. When in Rome . . .

The ladies who do things to you are very pretty, and Warwick and Alex were straining at the leash. I suggested that they had a massage, their nerve left them and they fled to the pool. Eileen had the works and she said it was a wonderful experience. She came out looking exactly the same as she went in, but she'd been caressed for three and a half hours and she said it was absolutely lovely, she'd never felt so relaxed.

Apart from the Recreation Centre and Roman Rooms, another refuge was a dress shop. Eating sweets or sticky buns was definitely out while trying on clothes, and it was encouraging to see my dress sizes going down, but I severely tested the patience of the shop assistants.

I had not been dieting very long, when one of my new ambitions were realized. I unknowingly made a conquest.

I went on a business trip with Warwick to America. Before we left we had lunch with a new business associate of Warwick's in London. The lunch was delicious and our host attentive. The prospect of the trip abroad (plus the good food and wine) had me sparkling and bubbling with good spirits.

Our host directed most of his conversation to me, and to my amazement phoned afterwards.

'You will want to speak to my husband,' I said.

'No,' he replied, 'to you, Belinda. When are we going to meet again?'

I was absolutely thrilled and could not wait to tell my husband. He, to my surprise, was not as thrilled as I was at my first proposition in years.

My instructions from Randal became rather erratic. He was travelling a great deal and his letters were taking a long time to reach me. I began to train myself. I discovered, however, that my method of running as fast as I could for as long as I could, interspersed with long walks, was not necessarily the best way.

In a transatlantic phone call to me, Randal told me that I had to run as slowly as I could and to forget about speed and 'personal bests'. The next day I went out and tried to run as slowly as I could for as long as I could – and made a breakthrough.

I was spending the weekend with my stepdaughter, Rachel Anderson, who lives in Southend. Rachel became a convert to running and now runs regularly, about 25 miles a week. At this time she was still only considering it, so I set off on an unfamiliar route on my own.

I concentrated on running slowly without worrying too much about distance, explored new roads and was shouted at by an irate farmer who did not like a fat lady running through his cabbage patch. I met a crocodile of small boys on a nature ramble who had a lot to say about a large lady jogging past them with big bouncing boobs and buttocks. I ran faster to get past them, but the taunts still floated along behind me. I was spurred to a much faster pace. I heard a yell of 'Shake them tits!' 'Look at her backside. Don't 'alf wobble.'

Finally I lost them, rounded a corner and settled down to a wheezing run, exhausted but still able to focus on my stop-watch. Thanks to those small boys and their lively sense of the ridiculous, I had run for twenty-five minutes, fifteen minutes longer than ever before.

From then on I knew I would be able to run a lot longer and further. Nearly six months after I began my walking/running regime I at last had become a proper runner.

Now that I was running properly, my regime was to change slightly. Randal told me I should do at least one long slow run/walk a week and to vary my runs in length and effort. For example:

Monday:	Walk/jog for ten minutes fast.
Tuesday:	Walk/jog for fifteen minutes slowly.
Wednesday:	Rest.
Thursday:	Walk/jog for fifteen minutes slowly and time it.
Friday:	Walk/jog for fifteen minutes fast and time it.
Saturday:	Walk for fifty minutes slowly.

Randal suggested I follow his example and give up drinking in a Moroccan sense. He had recently been to Morocco where they only classified spirits as an alcoholic beverage. Wines and beers were put in the same category as lemonade. It was an attractive form of hypocrisy and I became a Moroccan drinker, wine only, and cut down on the cigarettes.

Diary

Got mugged by a bottle of wine and a few strange cocktails and a dinner yesterday, my birthday of course. Today at Weight Watchers I hadn't lost anything and I've got a hangover and I'm fed up. Boozing really doesn't suit this slimming business and I'd thought I'd been so moderate. I resolve to give it up. Going to London tomorrow, I'll try not to eat until I return home.

Ran 2 miles, swam 25 lengths and walked 2 miles.

I had already discovered that drinking did not seriously affect my running (though a hangover seriously affects your desire to get out of a warm bed early in the morning and brave the elements in a skimpy tracksuit with cold rain pouring down the back of your neck and off your nose).

Cigarettes can set back training for weeks. At a party my resolve was weakened by the drinks and I started smoking. Maybe only four or five cigarettes, but that was enough to undo the good of a whole week's training. Was it really worth it? A few puffs to ruin a week of hard slogging. How absurd! I would give it up, but I could not until a strong motive took over, and I still had to find one.

Running had become central in my life. I dreaded the thought of getting up on a dark, cold wet day, to run 2 miles. The alternative, however, was to sit in the warm and dry and feel guilty.

One day I kept putting it off because of a light drizzle, but the feelings of guilt were so acute I had to promise myself I would be outside and running at 12 noon whatever happened. At 12 noon there was a thunderstorm and I discovered an interesting thing about track suits – they stretch when very wet.

I set off in the storm telling myself it served me right for not going earlier but, to my surprise, the sensation was not unpleasant, rather like running in a shower. The water was soft and warm, the air fresh and sweet. I saw birds and other animals looking out at me from their shelter under bushes. I set off down the road feeling rather foolish. Cars splashed past, often drenching me, the drivers doing surprised double takes at the sight of me running in a storm.

One car stopped and offered me a lift and self-consciously I refused, explaining I was taking exercise. It was raining so hard I was thankful I could hardly see the face of the driver, but I knew he eyed me very strangely.

I also found in the heavy rain that my tracksuit trousers were stretching, and soon I was sloshing along stepping on the trouser legs.

Then it got even more difficult. The weight of the water and my loss of weight meant that the trousers, which were already a little loose, were falling down. I tried to grab hold of my trousers with one hand, trying not to trip over my flapping trouser legs. My sleeves had also stretched and were flapping over my hands.

My feet were afloat, thumping down not on tarmac or rubber soles, but on water. I felt I was running under water. It was an uncomfortable and most undignified run, but it had one major advantage at the end when I checked my time. I had run 2½ miles in twenty-eight minutes, two-and-a-half minutes faster than ever before. The bad conditions spurred me on, there is no incentive to speed greater than an overwhelming desire to finish a run and get home to a nice hot bath. Motivation is everything.

The time had come, my trainer announced, for me to enter a Fun Run. Randal had selected a large Fun Run in Banbury near to where he lived for 10 October. I was rather apprehensive, but I was going to show the family what I had achieved.

7 Nearly the End

There was no hint of possible disaster as the time for my first public test, the 3½-mile Banbury Fun Run, arrived. After nearly five months of training, I was beginning to acquire some self-confidence.

I weighed 17 stone (down from 22 stone); nevertheless, the vast bulk was still there, only the outline had receded a little. I could tell the difference, but most people still saw me as massively overweight. I was going to be the fattest person in the Fun Run and, like most fat people, dreaded looking foolish, being conspicuous, drawing attention to myself. I also dreaded coming in last. Randal promised me this would not happen even if he had to carry me over the finishing line.

I also had to cope with my biggest problem – my bosom, which bounced up and down to cause both discomfort and embarrassment. When I ran my bra straps drooped down over the tops of my arms and pinned them down, so the first five or ten minutes were spent hoisting up my straps.

After a while they stayed put, due either to sweat, or to my muscles expanding. This was simply not good enough, it was really quite painful and occupied a great deal of my thoughts. Before the Fun Run I started to search for a suitable running bra for a lady with a size 50D cup bust. In the event I was not going to find a really suitable bra until I had slimmed down to a 38B, the largest size made in the Warner Athletic bra. Meanwhile, I made do with the firm-control bras from Marks and Spencer. It seems incredible now when I look at my old bras. I ask myself, how could my current, modest size 36B bust ever have got to a size so monstrous?

As the date for the Banbury Run approached I was assured it was a large race with lots of children, older people and beginners taking part, but I still felt I was going to make a fool of myself.

I would have to run 3½ miles. My last training run over that distance took forty-three minutes and was a struggle. My schedule was to wind down a week before the race, running less each day, and not at all two days before. Randal told me to stop drinking and smoking, but to have plenty of sex to help relax me and let me sleep properly.

Diary

9 October 1982
Yes, there *is* an improvement in my sex life!

For breakfast on the day of the run, we all ate a bowl of muesli, bran and banana, then wholemeal toast and delicious 'go faster' honey. We arrived at the sports hall in Banbury where the race was to start.

Diary

10 October 1982
All the family were out to watch Randal and me running this race. I collected my number from a desk and pinned it on the front of my bright pink T-shirt under my bust. I was told that only those with flat chests, or novices, pinned them over their busts. Some even put them on their backs

which was not considered 'correct'.

It was a brilliant October Sunday morning, thousands of people were milling about, there was an atmosphere of festive excitement.

Fun Runners are all shapes and sizes. Men and women, young and old, punks and county. There were svelte and stream-lined ones like thoroughbred racehorses, standing with controlled calm waiting for the start. There were cheerful housewives with borrowed tracksuits and their son's sneakers, out for a giggle and drinking tea from plastic cups.

One man was dressed as a parrot, some others as ballet dancers. One team was chained together as convicts. A man in a nightshirt was hand in hand with a girl dressed as a baby with an overlarge dummy in her mouth.

The 'Fun' part of the run certainly took hold. One woman was to run with a child in a pushchair, and a very old lady in a wheelchair was being pushed by a nurse. I saw a group of exquisite young men with carefully coiffured hair, make-up and ear-rings, and was told by my friend Jane that these were to be some of the front runners.

Everywhere people were limbering up. Some hard-eyed, hard-limbed ones had already done their preparations, others stretched their muscles, touched their toes, jumped up and down and chattered nervously. Someone lit a cigarette and a ripple ran through the crowd. I realized that, in all the thousands of people assembled, there seemed to be only one smoker.

All around people started to talk about smoking. I heard stories of famous athletes who smoked twenty a day, but these stories always ended with the observation: 'Think what they could do if they didn't smoke at all.'

Tension built up and suddenly I discovered that I had many ailments. I felt queasy with indigestion and a headache. Perhaps they were warning signs for flu. I wondered if I had twisted my ankle. Then the gun went off and we slowly surged forward, all hint of aches and pains forgotten in the panic of the start. The run itself was something of a blur. I was horrified as the main body of runners disappeared and in a matter of seconds the comforting mass of people had gone and I was left with the halt, the lame and the children, but everyone was happy and cheerful, if a little anxious.

I was puffing my heart out, convinced I would not finish. It was all so different from my usual 3½ miles round the Castle grounds where I know each turn and dip in the road. I fell further back all the time. The front runners were out of sight.

I felt I was the last runner, and probably the only runner as I trotted along the roads lined with friendly encouraging faces, not the least being the policemen holding up the traffic. Everyone was smiling cheerfully, were they just glad it was not them out there running? One middle-aged overweight woman leapt into the road as I went past and yelled at me, 'Go on gal – you can do it.' It gave me a tremendous boost and for the first time I thought to myself, 'Perhaps this is fun after all.'

All the vicars in town had promised to preach extra-long sermons so that the congregations did not spill out on to the course during the run, but it was difficult to believe there was anyone in church, the town was so full of people. I was so worried about coming last that I forgot about fatigue.

To my surprise, after a couple of miles, a lot of people were walking and I was still running. Slowly I began to overtake a few people; some of them seemed amazed to be overtaken by an enormous lady with a pink shirt, and they flashed past me again a few minutes later. When I thought the torture would never end, that I had been running for most of my early life, we entered the Recreation Field again, the finish line where we started. I was a long way behind but I was by no means last. I was very glad to see the end in sight but I was to learn that a race is not over until you cross the finishing line. I still had to do one circuit of the field, and waiting to spur me on was Randal and my stepdaughter Caroline. They both knew I did not want to be last, but did not know that there were still quite a few people behind me.

They decided to help me on, running on either side. Randal kept giving me encouraging pep talks, and I was aware that all the family were watching; there were also friends and a photographer. I desperately wanted to put on a last spurt to make my family cheer. Suddenly I was in trouble, and the finishing line seemed to recede into the distance. It was in fact only about 100 yards, but it seemed out of reach. My heart was thumping and my breath was painful. My body was screaming at me to stop.

Each breath seemed to come too late, my head was spinning, I could not see, and I felt I was going to collapse. My legs were wobbling and I had to concentrate to stay upright, putting one foot in front of the other. Then, from a long way off, I heard someone say, 'You've made it.' I saw Randal's worried face, he knew I was over the top. I had no idea where I was. I only knew I had an overwhelming urge to be sick.

Totally stunned, I stood in line to receive a card telling me I was 1,460 out of 1,500 runners. Well, at least there were a few behind me, mostly children, but I didn't mind. I had done it. I was thrilled, proud, satisfied, exhausted. Later I was to go into a decline, lying in bed alternately burning and shivering.

We went home and the ill, dazed, remote feeling continued. I crawled into bed and slept. When I woke up I felt dreadful, burning hot and shivering as though with a very high fever. I wondered if I had got flu. I was very depressed and disappointed with myself: such a feeble effort and such a pathetic reaction to go into a state of shock after a little run. I resolved to do my jogging in future round the lanes of Ringwood, but no more Fun Runs and certainly no marathon.

As I languished in bed burning and shivering, Randal and

Warwick arrived like the US Cavalry. I was brought back from the brink of a permanent decline by a large amount of champagne. I then got thoroughly into the spirit of the thing and dived into some bottles of Bulls Blood wine and proceeded to straighten out the whole family, whether they wanted it or not.

17 October 1982
It is now a week since my run and, in retrospect, I did enjoy the whole event. I am still very reluctant to repeat the experiment. I have been running slowly every other day and still feel guilty when I miss a day. But I'll never run a marathon.

8 Chomping and Cheating

I treated the Fun Run as a sort of triumph, but stopped making any references to a marathon which now seemed only a remote possibility.

I had been pushing myself for seven months and what had I got to show for it? Nearly 6 stone lost in weight, which sounded impressive, but 16½ stone made me the fattest runner around. No wonder I was almost last in the Fun Run and collapsed afterwards. In my diary I am not so sanguine about running.

Could we take a 'feel good' punishment pill which would stimulate the effect of running 10 miles? The bursting lungs, the streaming face, the blisters, the aching muscles, all got over in a few minutes like a Jekyll and Hyde potion. To run a marathon, 'Just take one pill an hour washed down with Gatorade and salt'?

After that run I found it so difficult to get started again on the training routine. I had keyed myself up for the Banbury Run, and given it everything I had. My diary entry for November says it all:

I ran a mile and nearly died. Everything is getting to me, booze, fags and people. I don't think I'll run again without help.

I did run again, of course, with the help of my family who

wanted me to succeed and my trainer, who still wrote, but not as often as before.

Diary

10 November 1982
Come on now Randal, wake up at the back. You don't expect me to keep on running with a trainer who is giving a good impersonation of the silent tomb. I believe I am much too slow. My ideal is the ten-minute mile as the basic running speed, and I am not improving. Surely I must go out for longer runs to show that I am breaking new ground, and get up my speeds on shorter runs. I have not run properly since the Fun Run. My legs creak as I move and if I bend down I am not sure I will get up again.

2 December 1982
I am a race horse that is severely off course. I have been stuffing myself with oats and bran, putting my nose out of the stable door, deciding it was chilly and putting it back again. I have been setting my stop-watch five minutes after I have started running and I have been finding excuses to stop halfway to give people directions, give advice to my husband (manfully trotting beside me), stop the postman for the post, inspect a new house that is being built, chat to dogs and coo over squirrels looking for nuts. It is incredible the number of diversions I can think of, even when I am out running, to slow me down or stop me.

I discovered little tricks (cheating) to improve my state of mind, my running and diet. It was a mistake, for example, to open the mail before going for a run. I would go downstairs to my letterbox, feeling bright and perky, and be hammered senseless by those long legal envelopes and those bossy little buff ones with windows. Trying to run after a bad mail is very difficult. Now I only open my mail after a run when I've had my bath and two cups of coffee, when I am feeling at my strongest and most optimistic!

The battle to lose weight remained the hardest struggle. I decided it was possible to cut out a lot of temptation by only tuning into BBC channels on television so as to avoid all those enticing commercials for food and drink.

Diary

I was awarded a silver donkey this week for being the best Weight Watcher during the month – I've lost 19 pounds. God knows what I'll do with the donkey, which is symbolic. It does not mean that you're an idiot to be there in the first place, neither is it the opinion of the slimming club of the idiots who pay over £2 a week to be weighed and told to eat less. The Award is a donkey with a bucket of water and a bundle of hay, which is all that donkeys need for sustenance – fatties take note.

I ate a lot of fruit and fibre: bran, apricots, prunes, baked potatoes, wholemeal bread, baked beans, lentils, fish, chicken, green vegetables and pulses generally. This way you absorb less calories and it also reduces the risk of cancer of the bowel. This diet also presents its own problems if you are running every day early in the morning as I was. Running stimulates the bodily functions so I had to be sure I went to the bathroom before I ran or, alternatively, carry toilet paper and run over a quiet route with plenty of bushes.

One quiet scenic route near my home was along a disused railway line. Apart from beautiful scenery and hedgerows, it afforded complete privacy. The railways which had once devoured and scarred the countryside, swallowing up beautiful land, were now giving back what they had taken.

As the lines were torn up, the hedgerows grew back and a treasury of flowers, plants and animal life grew up over the tracks. On my runs I discovered that disused railways are thriving communities of birds, rabbits, foxes and badgers and a riotous variety of wild flowers flourish secretly and undisturbed – a hidden nature reserve.

Meanwhile, I was always cheating myself. I knew a great deal of body weight is water. A strong diuretic taken a few hours before a weigh-in would produce a significant weight loss. To my shame I discovered a more effective and much more pleasant diuretic and that was booze. Two or three large vodkas or a bottle of wine a couple of hours before my weekly weigh-in at Weight Watchers, and I could lose as much as 5 pounds in weight.

The next day, of course, I was back to my old weight or more. When I eventually decided to cut out drinking alcohol entirely, however, I discovered an equally good way of shedding pounds in just an hour or two. I would go for a long run before a weekly weigh-in and be careful not to drink anything afterwards.

A 5-mile run showed a 2-pound loss and I later discovered a 10-13-mile run was good for 4 or 5 pounds weight loss. A good deal of the weight was back on again with a few cups of coffee, but there was none of the remorse of hangovers associated with the booze.

Diary

20 November 1982

Extensive research has brought me to the conclusion that thirst is nothing to do with exercise or sweating or needing water. The only thing that really makes you thirsty is drinking (booze of course) and eating anything, particularly curry. The less you eat the less you drink regardless of the amount of exercise in hot weather you take.

I reluctantly decided that drinking was not for me when I realized that my serious lapses usually started with a glass of wine. A few drinks and my good resolutions disintegrated. Drink would follow drink and then I would start eating. The next morning my remorse was pitiful. Self-disgust took over until I could think of nothing else. But, whatever happened, if one of my disciplines lapsed there was another to keep me on the track. So, as long as I was running, there was hope even if I was bingeing. If I stopped running, there was my diet.

I was beginning to bounce back, to recover some of my old optimism and confidence as Christmas loomed.

I was looking better, my skin had a glow and my husband said I shone in the dark. Of course he was exaggerating, but there is a fitness glow. Unfortunately, it is only an early reward; as you reach full fitness it seems to dim, or maybe you just get used to it.

I knew I was looking a good deal younger. At 16 stone my clothes were still shapeless tents, but my body seemed to know there was a future where everything was possible.

Then came a blow which threatened to jeopardize all my hopes.

I came back from one run with an ache in my knees. I thought little of it, but the next day I noticed that it was worse. I tried to ignore it, a big mistake: always listen to your body, especially when you are running, be aware of aches and pains and what your body is trying to tell you.

For three weeks I continued running, the pain in my knees getting more severe.

One day I was on my hands and knees sweeping the kitchen floor with a dustpan and brush. I put my hand to the work surface to heave myself on my feet. Nothing happened. I tried pulling myself up with two hands. Still nothing. My knees had gone on strike. They refused to function. Still on my hands and knees I crawled to the chair and table, and painfully I heaved myself with my arms on to the chair.

My legs were useless. I was on my stomach across the chair when Warwick came in. With his help I turned myself round and sat on the chair. He then held me under both arms and hauled me to my feet. I thanked God that my legs still supported me and walked gingerly out of the room.

After eight months of really heavyweight duty, my knees had had enough. I went straight to the doctor who told me to stop running and to forget forever my marathon.

'Your body is just too heavy for the strain you are putting on your joints,' he said. 'You have tried hard but now you have to pay the price.'

I made some distracted phone calls to Randal. He was a little more optimistic but still told me to prepare for the worst.

'Have a good rest, and then try again very, very carefully,' he added. 'But you might have to face it, love, the doctor may be right, you may just be asking too much of your knees.'

9 Reasons to Quit

Inside I felt so much fitter and stronger it was easy to forget I was still an incredibly fat person. My doctor was unmoved by my optimism. It was all very well, he told me, to feel different, but there was a long way to go before there was any real change, before I achieved normal weight. Meanwhile he advised me, 'Keep to a sensible diet, light exercise and walking. Swimming is always good, but forget about running for the time being.' It was not advice I wanted to hear, and my diary for a previous week reflected this.

Diary

When running today I improved my best time by five seconds. Read in the paper today that doctors say that jogging is bad for your muscles, and causes blood clots which could affect your heart, is bad for females and anyone over forty and children and teenagers, which doesn't really leave a lot of people. I can't believe that anything that makes you feel so good can be that bad for you. I am convinced that the alternative (no exercise and my old lifestyle) would kill me far quicker. I feel like a heavy Victorian chest which has been fixed with smooth castors – I just glide along now.

Bye for now – don't miss the next thrilling instalment. Will Belinda lose another pound in weight? Will she knock a whole second off her front-gate run? How many times will she weigh herself in the bathroom? Will her tracksuit survive another wash in the machine? And more – much more.

Although this extract revealed how boring running could be, and the medical problems, I was not prepared for the possibility of giving it up altogether. A friend warned me, 'Vanity can be very dangerous, Belinda. I never thought I would see you running after your youth.'

My mother, as usual, warned that I would do myself a serious injury. The consensus to give up running, to discipline my eating and lead a quiet life was unanimous. Perhaps I *had* left it too late. But how could I give it up when it made me feel so good? Surely I had just begun? But I had the memory of the Banbury Fun Run, where I ran myself into a state of collapse over 3½ miles. Perhaps I *should* give up.

Playing safe, as most people advised, was a comfortable option. Maybe I was motivated by vanity. I almost purred when my husband told me how pretty I looked. Then maybe I thought he was just saying that as encouragement. Training, after all, was a bed of nails.

My mother pointed out, quite accurately, that only a decade ago the 26-mile marathon was thought to be too mentally and physically stressful for even trained women athletes.

In the Olympics the marathon had only just been approved, as a woman's event, for the first time in the history of sport.

True, argued my mother, more people were running marathons than ever before, helped by modern dieting and training methods, but a woman in her mid-thirties who had never previously been interested in running or athletics, who was handicapped by carrying double her weight, who had just had a serious illness, had the odds very heavily stacked against her. Now with this knee trouble, surely the sensible thing to do was give up before I did myself permanent damage?

For three weeks I lumbered about the Castle, helped in and out of chairs. If a chair did not have arms or a handy helper, I was quite stuck. If I bent down, I was likely to tumble over and lie like a beetle on its back, unable to right myself without help. I was a fine example to proclaim to people, as I did, the benefits of running. I wondered if I was looking for an 'out'.

Then I got some marvellous letters from my friend Jane who insisted that everyone, including top-rank athletes, had setbacks, not just fat people. 'Go swimming instead of running until your joints are better,' she advised. 'Cut out road running, which jars the knees, in favour of cross country. But don't give up.'

Then Randal wrote to remind me of my original aims.

'You are like me,' he wrote, 'a hedonist, who puts the pursuit of pleasure as one of life's priorities. You are not just training for a marathon, you are getting yourself fit to catch up with and enjoy all the pleasures of life.'

I had to go along with that. I was jeopardizing more than just a 26-mile running ordeal. I also wanted to try so many new experiences: water skiing, windsurfing, scuba diving, squash, camping and mountain climbing.

In three weeks I lost 15 pounds. Five weeks after my first undignified collapse I was ready to run again. Carefully I ran along a grassy path. My knees held. I took it easy as Jane advised, as though I was a beginner again. She told me to run a mile, then walk a mile. I ran a mile and felt as though I had done nothing. Eight months after my first horrific, wheezing thirty-second run, I found a mile run did not make me sweat, and certainly was not tiring. What was I worrying about? I had come a long way.

My mother still worried that I might have a heart attack. My doctor and medical members of my family thought the marathon a step too far, but Warwick always supported me.

On one occasion out running, a neighbour stopped me.

'Don't you dare drop down dead outside my house,' she said with obvious agitation. 'My husband is not well and could not pick you up. Neither could I!'

I promised to try to collapse outside another house.

My new confidence made my work better. Out running I would sometimes get bright ideas, so I took a notebook and pen along with me, wrapping both in a polythene bag (sweating would make the paper soggy) and tucking them into my waistband.

My new positive attitude, a calmer frame of mind, helped me to face parties. I used to hate entering a room of strangers, talking to people I did not know. I thought I was an embarrassment to myself and my host. I dreaded Christmas, although I enjoyed our own family parties. I used to knock back drink to bolster my confidence. The following day I was not only hungover, but squirming with shame at the memory of outrageous things I had said and done. If my memory was occasionally selective, my teetotal husband used to fill in the details.

My first Christmas since I started running was the best for many years. On one party day I postponed my run until just before getting ready. As a result I had no need to down a few quick drinks beforehand and rediscovered the greatest gift of all for nervous party-goers – to be a very good listener.

As the party got under way I seemed to be one of the most popular people in the room. It probably helped that I was becoming well-known as the eccentric fattie who wanted to run a marathon. Running at much the same time every morning, usually when other people were on their way to work, I was seen by most of the neighbours.

My identification with the fitness cult was not altogether a boon for hostesses. The moment I entered a room, conversation switched exclusively to the subjects of weight, diet, fitness and running, and remained there until I left.

Apparent admiration was sometimes a trap. One woman gushed admiration, then regaled other guests with stories of how stupid and futile was my type of endeavour. She sounded so authoritative and looked so beautiful and fit herself, I was made to feel foolish. Nevertheless, the conversation returned to the original topic of me, my running and my diet.

One woman admitted to weighing 19½ stone. Sally was about my age and very pretty. Although it was our first meeting, she felt she could confide in me.

'I know I should go to my doctor, but I won't show him my bloated body,' she said. I sympathized with her and advised her to try running, really to have a go.

Later, someone came up to me. 'It is a shame about Sally,' they said. 'She is actually quite a nice woman.' I felt like hitting them, although they meant well. Then I realised that the patronizing talk about Sally, her fairground-freak status, was familiar stuff to me. I also realized, with some elation, that I was no longer considered to be in that 'poor thing' freak class. I was still a curiosity, but a socially acceptable one, in the fitness category. I left the party, determined to help other fatties like Sally.

As I happily bustled around with lists, wrapping paper and secret bundles, and did endless shopping, I reflected that the previous Christmas I had just emerged from my lonely room in the radiotherapy centre in Southampton General Hospital.

Those dark days were still fresh in my memory, when I lay flat on my back, my insides being slowly burned with radiation, terrified of moving in case the phial of radium packed inside my stomach contaminated other organs of my body.

The specialist had warned me that my 'cure' would cause temporary or permanent damage to bladder and bowels if the radiation was not contained within the womb. Lying alone in that hospital bed, I knew that if I survived the cancer I could still be permanently ill. I thought I would rather die than face a humiliating handicap.

My hospital check-ups had been reduced from monthly visits to six-monthly. My post-operative depressions were behind me. I had the running and the weight loss to thank for that and some very skilled nurses and doctors. I told myself that I owed it to them, to my family, to myself, to keep to my diet despite Christmas.

On one occasion, when the family had gone out for a walk, I sat down in front of the television with a large tin of chocolates. I intended to taste just one. When I heard my family returning, I had emptied the whole tin. I hid the evidence quickly and promised myself I would make amends with an extra fast run the following morning.

10 Finding It

Shortly after Christmas I experienced three firsts. I ran in my first snowstorm. I had my first case of 'numb bum' and my first 'runner's high' – yes, the real thing.

Thinking about the weather and the run is the worst part. Being there, facing the snow, ice, sleet, wind and rain is much more bearable than you imagine. Once you are accustomed to it, and that happens within minutes of going out, you enjoy yourself and wonder why you ever worried.

One difficulty, when you run in bad weather, is that motorists cannot believe anyone is stupid enough to brave the elements of their own free choice. They keep stopping to offer lifts, particularly if you are, like me, a non-athletic shape. The day I went running in a blizzard was no exception.

It was dark and overcast so I was wrapped warmly in my thickest tracksuit, a jacket with the hood up and gloves. The snow and wind started to hit me, the icy wind bit into my skin and took my breath away. Snowflakes settled on my eyelashes and melted into my eyes; soon I was almost blinded. The cold air seared the back of my throat and I could only open my eyes every five steps to see where I was going. Struggling against the wind was exhausting and occupied my energy and thoughts entirely. Ten minutes into the run felt like an hour, and as I pressed on I felt I had been running all my life.

The relief when I turned around for the homeward run was

immense, the wind droppped and I was smiling. The motorists stopped to ask if anything was wrong.

One driver reversed for 2 miles down a narrow lane to see if I was in trouble. I felt ungracious refusing such a gallant offer of help. He asked me if anything was wrong. I said I felt fine, but in fact was suffering a severe attack of 'numb bum'. When you are running in very cold weather and you put in a lot of extra energy, the heart and vital organs call for more blood to cope with this extra demand.

The body diverts some of the blood circulation from the extremities as extra fuel to pump round the heart. This causes a feeling of numbness in the buttocks, arms or legs. My husband told me that, in the cold, he sometimes felt as though his extremities would fall off! Nothing does fall off, of course, but numbed extremities do feel particularly uncomfortable.

One of my more interesting experiences that winter was to reach the 'runner's high' – the real thing, the 'peak experience' so often described to me by athletes as similar to a sexual orgasm.

On earlier runs I had felt happy and contented but I could not say it was anything more than a touch of euphoria due, some medics told me, to noradrenalin being released into the bloodstream.

One reason that running is addictive is that it gives you a good feeling, but the real 'runner's high' is something runners are coy about. It takes persuasive questioning to get firsthand information. I knew it was somewhere out there and I determined to see what it was like.

Bruce Tulloh, in his book *The Complete Jogger*, affirms that running really spikes up your sex life. Randal was uncharacteristically diffident on the subject. I wondered if it was really just a feeling of special fitness, or 'well-being' that came from running. Randal said he thought it was more than that, but would not develop the theme.

I asked my friend Jane, an experienced marathon runner. This time persistency paid off and I struck gold.

'Yes,' said Jane, 'running has its own reward. It gives you more than a feeling of accomplishment, of responding to and meeting a challenge. It is more like a sexual orgasm – an orgasm of the blood. I get it at the 15-mile mark, but I believe it varies for everyone.'

Jane, who has a science degree and is a notable athlete, was not given to exaggeration. Then the American sprinter and gold medallist Evelyn Ashford said, after her Olympic triumph, 'I get a feeling between space and time. I don't get it often, but when it's there it is better than having sex.'

Evelyn was a short-distance sprinter and I discovered she was right, you do not have to wait until the 15-mile mark, like Jane, before you experience a very positive sexual lift from running. This feeling, as Evelyn and Jane say, adds a lot to the pleasure of living.

That 'special feeling' was going to free me, give me a positive happy feeling, make me feel more desirable and confident, stop me thinking about what I wanted to eat. It made me think about something else I wanted to do!

I talked to everyone I could about the 'high'. After an initial shyness and embarrassment some were eloquent, describing the 'high' in terms of a 'born again' religious experience.

An athletics coach talked about the 'joy of the moment, when you are carried along and feel you can skim the fields and the trees. When your feet are like wings and your spirits soar.' Sounds like being weightless I thought, and this was from a 15-stone athletics coach whose days were spent in a gymnasium instructing strong silent men to lift weights.

One 18-stone weight lifter, whose usual conversation was about muscles and weights, spoke about the exquisite sensation of the warmth and well-being that flooded his body, past the pain barrier of strenuous exercise. 'I thrill to be alive and on this planet,' he said. He talked about a greater 'awareness'.

This was all very intriguing, so I did more research and consulted medical experts who, to my delight, confirmed that the 'runner's high' or 'peak experience' was known to them. They explained it as a hormonal change in the body, which triggered during extreme exercise enkaphalins and endorphins, a morphine-like compound, to be released into the brain. These compounds gave a climactic feeling of happiness and well-being. Yes, said my medics, intensive exercise does produce a drug-like, or sex-like 'high'. The compounds are also a potent painkiller which enables people to sustain extreme pain during exercise with bearable suffering.

Some doctors told me that the 'runner's high' could become addictive (goodie!) with runners suffering similar withdrawal symptoms as a drug addict if prevented from getting their 'fix' for several days. It could make them irritable, edgy, nauseous and shaking.

This was more or less how I used to feel every morning *before* I started running: the hangover, the raw nerves, the sickness, the jitters, the headaches. I felt that being hooked on running was going to do more good than my current addictions to booze, cigarettes and chocolate cake. Not only that, but with luck I would one day experience the 'real thing' the 'turn-on' for myself. Perhaps it would recharge my whole motivation.

If only I could experience the 'runner's high', the running would be a total substitute for a lot of the sins of the flesh – and a total health package. It could replace food, booze, sex and drugs! It could put the doctors out of business!

But the 'runner's high' eluded me for a long time. I began to wonder whether it was just myth, whether the doctors, my runner friends, even Jane, were having me on, or was I just a 'frigid runner'?

I got my first 'runner's high' experience during my first 9-mile run in February 1983. My usual run was now about 2½ miles with an occasional 4 miler thrown in.

I set out on the 9-mile route with my husband who was walking some of it to keep me company.

At the 5-mile mark I was still going strong. It was a beautiful day and I was skimming along. My whole body relaxed – and then it happened. A lovely warm feeling flooded through me, throughout my whole body. I felt I could jump off the earth and mingle with the clouds, be one with the trees and the sunshine. It was an ecstatic feeling, a feeling I never wanted to end. In an abstract way I felt myself running, my feet gently hitting the pavement without apparent stress or effort.

My mind seemed not entirely conscious, random thoughts floating in and out again. I felt I had to make no effort. I just drifted along, blissfully unaware of time or distance. Then my body took over and gradually I came down to earth and the reality of my breathing and my legs, now very heavy, pounding the pavement. My eyes were smarting and I felt very thirsty. I was beginning to feel I had run enough, but I ran on. I had two options: either I ran back home or I walked back home, and the walking would take longer and signify failure, so I ran.

I wanted to get home and had pleasant daydreams of a hot bath and coffee. Every run takes you through different thresholds or phases of pain. The last mile on this run was very long. I was counting each step, giving myself goals like the old days. If I can make it to the old oak tree, I then must just make it to the pillarbox, it's not that far then to my home.

I began counting the driveways to the houses. Three more houses, I thought, and then I'll have to stop. Then just three more. . . . Finally, I reached the Castle and home. My legs were wobbly, everything ached. Suddenly I remembered I had originally set out with Warwick and I hadn't see him for a very long time. I thought I'd better go and rescue him in the car; I could also check my mileage. I picked up the car keys and walked to my car. I could feel my joints stiffening.

I sat in the car and turned on the engine, but I could not see out. I was sitting in a thick fog of steam – the heat from my body, like a race horse after a hard gallop on a cold day. As fast as I quickly wiped the windows, they steamed up again. There was nothing for it but to wait until I had cooled down.

Eventually I found my poor bedraggled husband hobbling not far from home, and very pleased to get a lift the rest of the way. We measured our route and I had run exactly 9 miles. I felt very pleased with myself.

We arrived back and got out of the car. Then we were both really in trouble. Our bodies had seized up, I could almost hear my joints creaking, I thought I would never be able to straighten my body. Warwick was almost as bad.

Together, arm in arm, we staggered to our front door moaning audibly. Our neighbour, Malcolm Smith, stopped us, and asked if he could help, had there been an accident?

'It's nothing,' we said. 'We've been out enjoying ourselves on a run.' I heard Malcolm say in an undertone 'Rather you than me – must be mad.'

After a deep bath, a brisk rub-down, and a cup of coffee by an open fire, we felt a lot better. I looked out over the river idling past, the picture-postcard view of the snow-covered banks, and at Theo, my Birman cat, purring contentedly on my lap. I felt a tremendous sense of contentment and peacefulness.

'Can't wait to go on running tomorrow,' I said to Warwick. I was remembering the high.

Warwick looked at me proudly. 'You are a glutton for punishment, Belinda,' he said.

11 Danger Abroad

I was aware of the danger. I had been there before. I had travelled with my husband, flying from one country to another with all the attendant temptations; the break in routine and the excuse not to do anything physically demanding because of jet lag or fatigue. There was the dreadful temptation of 'room service' in hotels, of new exotic foods to be tasted and, apart from my husband, there was no one to see me breaking my rules.

This time, I told myself, would be different. I weighed myself at London Airport and, allowing for clothes, I was about 15 stone 3 pounds. We planned to be away for a month. First we had to go to the United States and then to Egypt. Would I survive the different temptations that these countries offered?

Both countries had their plusses and minuses for a running dieter. In America there were plenty of diet foods available wherever we went, no excuse not to stick to my diet – but there was also a lot of pressure to eat absolutely delicious, attractively presented, high-calorie foods.

Americans seem to be divided into two camps: those who are very health conscious and determined to stay young, slim and vital for as long as possible, and those who have succumbed to the marvellous food advertisements on television, radio, newspapers and roadside hoardings.

Food is also quickly available in the United States twenty-four hours a day from delicatessens, drug stores and thousands of fast-food restaurants, as well as from a dazzling array of high-class gourmet restaurants. You are surrounded by advertisements of beautiful people on billboards and television, eating beautiful food. Food is shown as a way of loving and caring. Single portions in restaurants are enough for four people. So normal is abnormal that people, grotesquely fat like me, are not unusual.

Our first stop was for three days in St Louis, Missouri. I had never been there before and Warwick warned me it was packed with good restaurants and would be a test of my resolution to keep to my running and dieting. I started off well.

Diary

22 February 1982

St Louis, Miss. Running along the riverfront below the magnificent St Louis arch which dominates the skyline so majestically by the water's edge. The weather was icy cold, a very marked contrast to the heated hotels, cars and subways. Nose, ears and fingertips froze as soon as we hit the outside. The air is so cold it leaves you breathless. Running along the waterfront from the hotel, Warwick and I were the only humans moving, the prospect was desolate. The only beings on earth? Is this what it would be like after the 'big one' dropped? The arch changes shape as you get closer. It becomes a hoop, a triangle, a curve, shooting towards the sky. It loses its fragile appearance to become disappointingly solid, a thing of concrete blocks, graffiti and iron railings. We ran around the arch twice, about two miles. Every part of my body became numb with the cold. Warwick looked rather blue and said that he was going back as one part of his body was about to drop off!

I carried on for a little longer, along to the road and to the museum. A cleaner was opening up there. She had a look of pure astonishment on her face as I ran past her. To make sure she had not imagined me, she stood out by the freezing road to make sure. The last half mile back to the hotel, the cold had entered my soul. I fell into the warm bright lobby, feeling like Scott of the Antarctic making it back to civilization. I expected people to stare at me in the lobby, which they did, but nothing was said. After all they have seen most things in St Louis.

We flew from St Louis to the sunshine of California where it is considered strange to walk anywhere. US cops will stop you and ask for your identity if you walk down a suburban street in the evening. The only people in Beverly Hills out walking were other Brits.

Running is different. Everybody runs in Beverly Hills. I particularly enjoyed running in the area of the movie stars' homes.

On one occasion a familiar figure swathed in a tracksuit, with hood and gloves, ran very fast past me. He looked remarkably like Ryan O'Neal. That is who he was. Seconds later his two bodyguards with two-way walkie-talkies ran past. This was a real sign of the times for America and a long way from my home in rural Hampshire.

Although no one walks in America there is a running rush hour between 5 and 6 p.m. in the evening. The sidewalks are so crowded with runners you have to signal to overtake. Hotels have circuits alongside the mandatory pool and jacuzzi. Early in the morning, I joined the others at the Ambassador Hotel, Los Angeles, as they pounded around a quarter mile wooden track, built specially for the purpose.

Diary

We are in Los Angeles and we are shattered. Have spent a couple of days running and swimming. There is a running track at the hotel and a lot of people use it. Could you believe a running track getting congested? I was very pleased that I was easily outrunning nearly everyone on the track. I was not always faster, but I jogged for much longer. I was surprised I did so well as there are so many joggers in LA. I found I was getting very satisfied with myself after only a comparatively short thirty-minute run. Few joggers at the hotel did it for more than fifteen minutes.

From Los Angeles we flew to Palm Springs to stay with friends, Harrison Price and his wife, Annie, at their luxurious home.

Our host's idea of exercise was to help the pool maintenance man scoop out leaves before his first extra-dry martini of the day. It was a real rest and I lay back and enjoyed the comfort.

Diary

Palm Springs is all right. I don't think I have slept so much in weeks. I've been lying under a star-studded sky in a warm bubbling jacuzzi with a glass of champagne in my hand. I have begun to feel human again – and then Warwick reads in the local paper that there is a Fun Run on the next day in the town starting at 6.30 a.m.

Warwick hustled me off to register and attend a pre-run lecture and surgery arranged by the organizers. The lecture was to warn runners of the problems they might have, and a doctor is available to discuss leg injuries and running ailments. It is all very serious, not a bit like the rather dotty Banbury Fun Run. . .

I ran the Palm Springs Fun Run 5 kilometres in thirty-two minutes. I had planned to run faster at the end, but chickened out when I remembered what happened when I speeded up in Banbury. It was difficult running in the very dry heat which, in the middle of a British winter, I had not really become accustomed to. The atmosphere is tense, and everyone looks very intent. I did surprisingly better than I expected against some rather impressive opponents, nearly all young and slim, with no children, and few runners over the age of forty-five. Out of the 250 entrants I came about 200; for me to run faster than fifty other young, apparently fit people was truly amazing.

We finished our American travels in the port of Tampa, Florida, 80 miles from Disney World. In the hotel there were maps of the 5-mile course round the waterfront of Tampa; this made it easier for me to keep to a routine. It is an old bicycle track, with exercise stations every few hundred yards.

Diary

10 March 1983
The exercise station was a sign on which there was a diagram of an exercise, beside a dismantled park bench which I think was meant to aid the exerciser. No one seemed to take any notice of them although there were plenty of joggers. The main trouble with the course was the uneven paving stones. On the way back I tripped and fell heavily (someone of over 15 stone does not fall lightly). This was something I had been dreading ever since I started running and in a way it laid a ghost, because I was shaken but unhurt apart from grazed knees, and I am sure I will run with more confidence now.

There seemed a lot more runners in Florida than California, which was surprising because the people here are immensely fat. Warwick and I are quite modest compared to most. I would say one in three people is overweight and one in five absolutely grotesque.

I found that our next stop, Egypt, was also a country which has a great many overweight people, and where I therefore did not feel out of place. My weight did not warrant a second glance in Egypt, where 15 stone must be considered almost normal for the average woman of my age!

Nearly all Egyptians are overweight, particularly women over the age of twenty-one. The custom in Egypt is for a pregnant woman to eat as much as she can. She gets fat with the first baby, and stays like that, with the weight gradually increasing as she stokes up for subsequent babies.

The staple food of many Egyptians living in Cairo seems to be very sweet and sickly cakes, washed down with cokes or syrupy mint tea. It is surprisingly difficult to get fresh fruit and vegetables in a country which is famous for growing both. Even good hotels are reluctant to serve a salad, and the food is heavy and rather greasy although, of course, there are exceptions. I have eaten delicious, if rather high-calorie, meals in people's homes. The Egyptian lentil soup is really a treat.

Though I found it very difficult dieting in America it was comparatively easy in Egypt where there is less temptation from advertisements and easily available food. The problem only lies with the lack of availability of suitable diet foods. The main trouble in Egypt was the running.

Egyptians are not used to large blonde ladies running around their ancient streets. Because of the heat, it is considered very strange to see anyone running. I was told that a running figure would automatically be associated with a crime. Egyptian women, of course, would never do anything so undignified.

I must have looked very strange. The trousers I had brought were now too big and fell down when I ran. Because it was so hot I wore my last year's summer clothes, all of them billowing, too big, and hanging like vast tents. On my feet I wore trainers.

The streets of Cairo are very crowded, so first I jogged around the shopping square attached to the Nile Hilton Hotel. It was about a quarter of a mile.

The first day I went for a run, the man washing the pavement dropped both his mop and bucket in amazement. Another man asked if anything was wrong. All the shopkeepers around the square came to the doors of their shops to look at this phenomenon. The square was hot underfoot and seemed endless – the sun was beating down. I was very embarrassed so I ran as fast as I could to get it over. Soon a crowd gathered to enjoy the spectacle. I ran with my heart pounding and the heat rising in my body like a pressure cooker. When I dived thankfully back into the air-conditioned hotel I looked down and found I was standing in a pool of water as the sweat literally poured off my body.

That experience was unnerving so the next day I tried running through the centre of the city. This caused a traffic jam so the next day it was back to my hotel circuit and the audience of interested spectators.

Diary

I am still not causing alarm and despondency and frightening the donkeys by baring my legs and wearing a T-shirt and shorts. I am still running in my ballooning dresses and would give anything for a track suit that fitted.

I am beginning to resemble a bumble bee in appearance. My legs have got thin, particularly the thighs which are now almost normal. My arms are also slimming down, the rest of me is still round and squashy.

Discovered the Gizeira Club. Quite daunting negotiating the road and bridges to get there, but worth it. We went at Ifter (the breaking of a religious fast during Ramadan) and found the Olympic pool virtually empty. Swam happily and then decided to jog round a field. It was very wet, the hosepipe was left on all the time, and full of potholes. It attacked me, ricked my ankle and soaked me. I could not manage all four sides as it was like an obstacle course with cats, kids, bicycles and Egyptian joggers all trying to trip me up. Foolishly I was wearing my trousers which, of course, kept falling down.

A word about Egyptian joggers. There are a few in the Gizeira Club, but they make allowances for the heat. They look very smart in their Nike tracksuits and shoes, but they do not actually jog, they walk. They have a dedicated, purposeful air, and are probably doing the most sensible form of exercise in a country with these weather conditions.

Weighed myself yesterday on the Nile Hilton Health Club scales. At first I tried to weigh myself on the men's scales and got thrown out by a furious attendant. I hunted around until I found the scales which women were allowed to use. To my horror I had apparently gained 2 pounds.

I am still running round the Nile Hilton square, have increased my time per lap by twenty seconds but am only doing two laps (about ½ mile). People expect to see me running and I have got used to my audience.

When I appear in the square, the hotel porter settles back in his seat to get comfortable. The cleaners stop chatting and lean on their brooms, there is a buzz of expectancy and excitement, as when the orchestra strikes up the overture before the curtain goes up. One shopkeeper has appointed himself my time-keeper, and sits importantly in his doorway with a big stop-watch. The illegal money changers cluster in the corner of the square, gullible tourists forgotten for a few minutes. Nobody seems inclined to join me, but then nobody laughs or makes fun. I am one of the sights of Cairo and I am there to be looked at and enjoyed, like the pyramids, or a really good dog fight. I will certainly be missed when I leave.

As I walk away from my running track along the streets the sounds of Cairo jostle in my ears: the eternal hooting of the traffic, the chants 'Change money', 'Very nice', 'Welcome', 'See my shop', 'No charge for looking,' 'I'm waiting for you,' 'Taxi, lady,' 'Pyramids very cheap.' Then I get the more obscure, 'Nice, nice, jumpy, jumpy,' and the forthright, 'Big bosom Missus.'

Sunday

At Magawish on the Egyptian Red Sea. A different world. A breeze made it cool and fresh but with 90° dry heat in contrast to the very humid Cairo. We flew to Luxor, the Valley of the Kings. There was only one plane a week to Magawish, Hurghada, so we decided to drive through the mountains of the Eastern desert, a wild, wild drive.

We arrived at a hotel in Magawish. I ran for ten minutes. Not easy on soft sand and heat of 87°. There is a lot of walking as everything is spread out, the chalet, the restaurant, the beaches and boats. A round trip is at least a 20 minutes' brisk walk.

The last time I was here I was very fat and ill and I sat firmly by the restaurant in the main area as I couldn't face all that walking about. Now I'm trying all the water sports. Got absolutely whacked after a day's snorkeling, the sun burnt my back which I left exposed on the surface of the water.

Quite a lot of runners, but then this is an athletic, sporty place. Snorkeling, windsurfing, sailing, archery, scuba diving, tennis and eating.

Unfortunately the food is quite good . . . .

We returned home to England via Cairo. Our friends Professor Khishin and his family gave a party for us. They had all heard about my ambition to lose weight and run a marathon, and were very encouraging. The meal they gave us was delicious.

When I returned home to England, I weighed myself on the scales. My fears were groundless, I had actually lost a pound, not much, but it was a sort of triumph when I thought how bad it could have been.

12 Suddenly One Summer

Back home and summer had come and I was running about 20 miles a week and slowly improving, my weight down to 14 stone 5 pounds. I had a tremendous day when I discovered I was a 'normal' size 18 – the first time for many years. No more looking in outsize-dress shops! Almost any store could fit me.

I was still much too fat, but I no longer felt fat. I began to feel lively and attractive, able again to wear fashionable clothes. But a photograph of myself at that time still showed me looking very overweight.

In fact I was feeling over-confident and the desire to keep on losing weight was not as strong as it should have been. So confident had I become, I decided to put aside my tracksuit and inhibitions and try running in a pair of shorts. I prepared for my shorts' debut with a couple of sunbed sessions to tan my legs a little. Then I bought the most flattering shorts I could find.

I was still self-conscious about the fat wobble around my thighs and knees, but an unsuspecting world seemed to accept my bare legs with uncritical indifference. Indeed, nobody appeared to give them a second glance – a pointer that I still had a long way to go.

But I did feel wonderfully free, running with bare legs.

Not long after I had bared my legs there was a pleasant new development to my life. A van drew up beside me while I was out running, and stopped. The driver apologized for interrupting me and asked about my running. He said he was seriously thinking of taking it up himself. Could I advise him about starting? Was weight a factor? How far should he run?

I was prompted into a thoughtful assessment of the benefits of running in relation to weight loss, a cure for depression, a way of toning up muscles and controlling hunger. There seemed to be no stopping my flow of information. Then he asked me if I was on holiday. No? What was I doing that evening? I had not suspected that his interest was just a pick-up line. It had been so long since I had been chatted up by a stranger that I had forgotten what it was like.

I ran on feeling foolish, but just a little flattered. The next day at the hairdresser it happened again. The only time I go to the hairdresser is about twice a year to have my hair cut. I choose a hairdresser entirely at random, depending on my mood and available time. I was exploring some back-streets in Bournemouth and stumbled across a tiny hairdresser which did not look as though it had an age limit (some hairdressers seem to discourage any customer over the age of twenty-five). I was attended to immediately by the proprietor, a man in his early forties who had obviously seen, and never forgotten, Warren Beatty in the film *Shampoo*.

He sat on a little stool on wheels and whizzed around me, staring hard at my face and issuing instructions all the while to his staff. He took enormous trouble over my hair although it was not a very exacting task. He leaned on my shoulders and caressed the back of my neck with his fingers. Where did I live? What was I doing that evening? He was not easily put off, and once again I felt a little foolish but flattered.

My diary records that 26 July 1983 was a red-letter day: the first time my bra straps felt really comfortable. One of the penalties of being overweight and top-heavy is the pain and bleeding when running, caused by chaffing bra straps. At that time I had gone from a massive size 50D to a 40C cup.

71

I was very pleased with myself until I met Valerie Viggars. I first noticed a plumpish, fortyish lady running along the lanes a little in front of me. I was thrilled to see her because I thought I might have inspired her to run. She was obviously local and therefore was probably following my example. I wanted to congratulate her, to encourage her and invite her to run with me, to tell her that running has its own reward. In short I wanted to be unbearably patronizing. All I had to do was catch her up.

To my chagrin the distance between us did not lessen. I ran faster, shaking my head over 'amateurs' who start with a flashy fast run only to collapse exhausted after a few hundred yards. We rounded the corner together. First Valerie, then Belinda. I was now running flat out, no longer chasing her for a little chat, it was my self-respect as a runner I was after. The gap between us widened. I was in trouble, my breathing was in gasps, my legs turning to jelly. Then she did a spurt and disappeared from view. I ran slowly home, a chastened, wiser runner.

Later on I met and made friends with Valerie. She spent hours helping me to train, running with me to improve my speeds but it took a long time before I could run as fast as Valerie. Then a leg injury held her back and I overtook her.

If I was too satisfied with my progress maybe I could blame the optimism which came with the lovely, attractive clothes I could now wear and the new sports – windsurfing and sub aqua – that I was trying. I was not losing much weight, but I was keeping stable with summer salads and a 5-mile-a-day run. I was so contented I would not have progressed any further if it had not been for a sea-urchin which stopped me running, and a 5 to 1 chance that got me going again.

13 Saved by Television

When I entered for the London Marathon I knew the chance of being accepted (particularly for a beginner) was about 5 to 1 against. Nevertheless I filled in the forms and sent them off with my £6 registration fee and promptly forgot all about it. That was in September and the marathon was not to be run until 13 May the following year, a comfortable eight months away.

I went on holiday to Eilat on the Red Sea coast of Israel. The second day there I trod on a sea-urchin when I was learning to windsurf, and hurt my foot. The only treatment was rest. So my four weeks in Israel were spent mostly on my back on the beach. The evenings were a problem; the sun set early and there was no night-life or entertainment. It was either early to bed or a long leisurely dinner.

Some Eilat restaurants were good and I think we ate in every one. For the first time in nearly two years I ate whatever I liked and was not running. I felt fabulous, on top form, so I did not worry. It was glorious to be free of my work and diet regime, although at the back of my mind I knew I would have to pay for my self-indulgence when I got home.

Already I noticed that my taste in food had altered. The big steak and chips and large smelly curries did not appeal like they used to do. The more subtle Chinese and French cooking appealed to me more. I ate too much, too often.

When I left for Israel my weight was just under 14 stone. When

I returned home I straightaway stood on the scales. I was nearly 15½ stone. Familiar remorse engulfed me, but that was only the beginning of my problems. Waiting for me was my acceptance for the London Marathon. I had virtually forgotten about it.

'Congratulations,' I read. 'The computer's electrical heart has been kind to you and picked you as one of those accepted for the London Marathon to be run on May 13th.' The acceptance letter went on to say how 'lucky' I was as there had been over 100,000 applications for 20,000 places.

I did not feel lucky. Condolences would have been more appropriate. Stunned by the enormity of the folly of my application I wandered around in a daze.

My husband was thrilled with the news, he wanted to phone all the papers and alert the television station. I was not in such a rush. I hid the phone book! I also asked him to wait before talking to anyone as I wanted to think it over.

I climbed on the scales again. Even with shuffling about, the needle still read 15 stone 7 pounds. I felt sick at my backsliding in Israel, at the months of wasted effort. I also knew that unless I did something drastic, panic would drive me to comfort eating and I would soon be back where I started.

I had recently put a television format to Television South suggesting a running and diet segment as a regular part of the sports programme. I had told them I had started to run and hoped to compete in the London Marathon. Mark Sharman, the Head of TVS Sport, and Vic Wakeling, the Programme Editor, had suggested I contact them if I had anything special to report on the marathon running scene. My acceptance for the London Marathon was special news, they might consider it qualified for the theatre of the absurd. I phoned and got an immediate response.

It was only a few days before Christmas but a TVS unit would be round to the Castle to film me, they said. It would be the first of a series of programmes for the Friday Sports Show on TVS.

If the news of my acceptance for the Marathon had thrown me off balance the imminent arrival of the television crew meant there was no turning back. No more backsliding or I would make a public exhibition of myself. I would be doing that anyway, but to expose myself as too weak for my own good would be humiliating. People would probably laugh at the idea of me running a marathon in any event. But why not me? This was my chance to escape once and for all from my old flab-ridden world, and to do so in front of the cameras. Maybe it would help me, a powerful monitor to prevent backsliding. I might even give hope to the thousands of others, who were the victims of their own ravenous appetites; who were obese and hopeless.

That night I dreamed that the television crew arrived and said they wanted to film me running along the road to prove I could really run. When I tried my legs were too heavy to move. In my dream my husband and friends tried to push me but I was rooted to the spot. I begged the camera crew to wait, that this had never happened before. I made a frenzied effort to move my feet. 'Hopeless, bloody hopeless,' said one of the crew, and then he and the others in my dream danced around me shouting, 'Fraud, fraud, fraud.'

In the morning I had rings under my eyes and was jittery. It was just as well that Warwick took control and put the house in order while I tried to compose myself and apply make-up.

The first arrival was a good-looking young man called Dave Bobbin. He introduced himself as the TVS reporter who would be interviewing me. He confessed with endearing frankness that he would need a coffee before he could face the day. He looked as though he was feeling the effects of a heavy party the night before; he was certainly not feeling strong enough to expose anyone as a fraud! Then six more men and a girl arrived. It seemed a large crew and I hoped they would think it was worthwhile.

They decided to film me in the kitchen, drawing-room and

bathroom, pristine as a result of my husband's hard work.

The crew were unhurried and professional. They were also friendly so I began to relax and enjoy the experience. I hoped very much that they were not going to do a 'poor soul' story: a pathetic fattie with an impossible pipe-dream.

The biggest bonus of all was being the centre of attention for five solid hours.

They filmed me on the bathroom scales, preparing a meal in the kitchen, sitting talking in the living-room and running along the road. While this was happening they laughed at my jokes and apparently listened to my slightest comment. After years of unimportance and invisibility, it was a heady experience.

Then suddenly it was all over. They finished the filming and, as I served drinks, they settled down to talk about Christmas plans and their own affairs. The spotlight was no longer on me and I tried hard to recapture it. 'I can run in the snow,' I said desperately. 'I can run in thunderstorms and on one leg.' But it was over, I resolved to be interesting enough in future to attract more television attention. Meanwhile I had to go back to being interested in other people. I wondered if everybody felt as I did after being filmed or whether I had a special case of the 'vanities'.

I regressed to childhood when the moment arrived to watch the result of the filming. I sat on the edge of my chair with a cushion over my face. But curiosity got the better and I peeped out. The programme was a great deal better than I had expected. They had accepted what I was doing and treated me gallantly, suggesting my attempt on the Marathon was courageous, although I am not sure I will forgive the director for those bottom-wobbling shots of me running up the steps of the Castle.

While the programme was still on the air, my telephone started ringing. Everybody I had ever known must have seen it. They were delighted I looked so well but most of them were astonished, even incredulous, at my ambition to run the Marathon.

The next day in the town, people came up to me and wished me well. I got free carrier bags for my shopping and the bank clerk did not look up my account on the computer when I presented a cheque for cashing. He just smilingly handed over the money. I was given a reduction in my taxi fares, I got served out of turn in a shopping queue, shopkeepers did not always want to see my cheque card when paying by cheque and I got served with great ceremony in restaurants. Dozens of women stopped me to tell me about their operations. I also heard some amazing stories of what some people had done to overcome or cope with their health problems. Sometimes I got a hint of 'my operation was worse than yours' but most people rightly thought I would be interested, although I soon got to the point where I felt I would scream if I heard the details of yet one more hysterectomy. A number of overweight women and men told me I was an inspiration to them.

People phoned me, wrote to me and stopped me in the streets. They wished me well and urged me not to give up. They asked my advice, but above all they left me in no doubt that I was no longer running just for myself. There was now the goldfish bowl of television to consider. I had to do something dramatic to offset my backsliding in Eilat and show significant progress before the next television programme went out.

I decided to give up drink and smoking. If I smoked as little as five cigarettes in an evening it put my training back a whole week. I tended to smoke when I had a drink, one sparked off the other, so it was best to cut them both out. Not necessarily forever, but until I had lost enough weight and was fit enough to run a marathon.

14 Enter a Stranger

Television introduced me to Tony Drinkwater, my new trainer, who was to play a key part in my next stage of training.

The introduction was brought about by an acute case of second thoughts by Television South, and a kind offer of help from Don Howard, the owner of the Olympian Health and Fitness Studio in Bournemouth.

My television programme sparked off a big response from viewers. Could a 15-stone, not-so-young housewife ever become fit enough to run a marathon? Wouldn't she collapse or do herself a permanent injury in the attempt? The possibility of my making a public spectacle of myself, a laughing stock, existed. I did not underestimate the degree of personal dedication and endurance that was required, but suspected that the television company questioned the wisdom of encouraging such an overweight lady as myself to put herself at risk in a marathon. They decided to put me into professional hands. They could then more responsibly make some lively programmes with a cliff-hanging finale – the Marathon itself.

To see I would be properly trained they took me to· the Olympian Health and Fitness Studio, where Don Howard and his wife Mary made me welcome and introduced me to Tony Drinkwater, my trainer. He was the manager of the gymnasium, and his vivacious wife Muriel ran their own health and beauty clinic, Studio Olympus, in Christchurch. They were both to help me a great deal, Tony with the actual training and Muriel with toning up the loose skin.

Tony was a forty-two-year-old athletics coach who had learned his trade while training recruits in the Royal Air Force. He was slim, tall, broad-shouldered, but surprisingly agile for a big man. He radiated vitality and enthusiasm and clearly knew a thing or two about physical fitness. He believed in weight training for running and he and his wife thought that their particular form of vegetarian diet was worth trying.

I still shudder when I watch the video of the first television programme showing me working under Tony's guidance: the mound of flesh quivering under the unaccustomed weights; my vast bosom heaving as I do a bench press; the total body wobbling as I jump up and down with the weights. Then I watched myself being weighed and measured. Vital statistics 44, 34, 44, weight 15 stone 3 pounds.

I was at first very sceptical about the benefits of the gymnasium.

'You are a very determined lady,' Tony said to me, 'but that alone is not enough. You have an awful lot to do and very little time. You will never make an athlete but, with a great deal of hard work, you might run a marathon. First I want you to shed at least 5 stone in weight. At the same time we have to build up your stamina to take you over 26 miles.

'This is not going to be easy but it is possible,' he said. 'The top part of your body, in particular, needs a lot of work, and we should improve your breathing.

'You do have a special thing going for you. Your resting pulse rate is very low and strong at 40. This is quite unusual and is found in some of the best athletes. Most people have a 60-plus pulse rate. It is something you are born with, although you can lower your pulse rate with exercise. You are in good company, Mohammed Ali, Sebastian Coe and Steve Ovett all have very low resting pulse rates.'

In his first pep talk Tony had accomplished an interesting double. He had made me very aware of the amount of hard work I had to put in, but he also made me believe that it was possible, and that I was something special. Later I was to find that Tony was not only a good talker and very kind but also the best listener I had ever met.

I did not at first feel comfortable in the gymnasium, however. I felt out of place surrounded by beefy, intense young men and lithe, graceful and equally intense young girls. Tony sensed my shyness and used to take me upstairs to a private room for workouts. Watching myself in the mirrored walls I thought how ridiculous I looked beside my slim instructor, I could not escape the reflection and I became even more determined to work harder.

I did not want to look ridiculous beside my instructor or anybody else in the gym; facing up to the reality of my obese shape before those relentless mirrors was an important stepping stone. I could not stand alone and carefully pose myself to advantage as I did with my mirror at home. At the gym there was always someone 'normal' to compare with and there was a high standard of physical fitness around me.

Tony put me on a light ten-day vegetarian diet. This included a substance called Spirulina, a high-protein form of seaweed or micro algae, found on a salt-water lake in Mexico, rather like a green scum, not very appetizing, but very nourishing and with almost no calories. I took six pills a day with meals. He also gave me potassium pills to replace the minerals and salts I lost through sweating while training.

Day One   Three small fruit meals.

Breakfast: 2 Spirulina, 1 potassium, 1 multivitamin
              pills. Grilled tomatoes on toast.
              orange, lemon and apple.

| Lunch: | 2 Spirulina, ½ melon, small fruit salad, tea. |
| Dinner: | 2 Spirulina, ½ melon, small fruit salad. |

| Day Two | Normal vegetarian day. Low fat, low carbohydrate, high protein. |

Breakfast:	2 Spirulina, 1 multivitamin, 1 potassium pills. Small bowl of unsweetened cereal with skimmed milk, or poached eggs.
Lunch:	2 Spirulina. Cottage cheese and green salad, fruit
Dinner:	2 Spirulina. Grilled white fish and steamed green vegetables or salad and fruit

| Day Three: | Vegetable-only day |

Breakfast:	2 Spirulina, 1 potassium, 1 multivitamin pill. Grilled tomatoes on toast.
Lunch:	2 Spirulina, green salad
Dinner:	2 Spirulina. Steamed courgettes, tomatoes, onions, peppers, celery.

Then back to a 'normal' fourth day of a vegetarian diet, then a fruit-only day and so on, until I had completed the ten days.

On the fourth day I felt absolutely dreadful – weak and ill with a foul taste in my mouth and a headache. But I dragged myself to the gymnasium and Tony reassured me that my reaction was perfectly natural. He explained that all the toxins were leaving my body.

On the sixth day I was beginning to feel a little better and not at all hungry. By the ninth and tenth days I was beginning to get rather bored with it all, but I was feeling terrific and had lost ten pounds in weight.

On the last day of the diet, I was to have a treat. A delicious fruit-and-vegetable salad with yoghurt three times. This was extremely pleasant and acted as a diuretic, flushing out any impurities left in the body.

This last day's diet was to become my standard diet for the rest of the time up to my marathon. For the next five months I would eat fruit, vegetables and a little natural yoghurt only for one day, followed by a 'normal' eating day of a low-fat, low-carbohydrate diet.

Tony recommended that I stop drinking coffee and drink only weak tea. I tried this for a while but decided that coffee was more satisfying for an empty tum. I did, however, drink only decaffeinated coffee to stop the jumpy feeling I got when drinking ordinary coffee.

Tony then gave me a set of exercises; at first without weights, then with weights as I became fitter. At first I practised alone with Tony, but as I became bolder and more confident I worked in the gymnasium where, to my surprise, I was completely ignored. Weight training is an absorbing hobby which requires a lot of physical effort and mental concentration. Everyone working out was too preoccupied with their own training to bother with me. In the past I had complained about invisibility, now I welcomed it.

I was easily the fattest there, but apart from the encouraging smiles from Don and Mary, Harry and Tanya, Shaleen and the rest of the staff, the occupants left me to myself. For their kindness and courtesy I was, and am, still profoundly grateful.

At first I thought I would never get the hang of the exercise routines. Everybody else seemed to manage them so easily, while I struggled with the simplest knee bend or push up. But I progressed faster with the weight training than with anything else. In only one week, working out three afternoons a week, I managed a whole forty-minute routine, involving bench press, lat pulls, pull overs, squat thrusts and so on.

I found I was able to lift weights which only seven days before had been impossible. I also learned poise and balance so I didn't fall over when doing a squat jump or a leg thrust.

My life changed. Tony told me that to succeed I had to be selfish. Nothing must come before my training and the gymnasium. My husband and family agreed.

I must say I soon became very used to being 'number one'. I totally committed myself to a life of selfishness for the next five months (the price of success), to live, work and think only about one person. This meant, for example, that I only cooked food for my family if I could eat myself. Meals were mostly not cooked at all as they were fresh fruit or salad. If the family wanted anything else they had to buy and prepare it themselves.

The safest place of all was the Olympian Studio where there was no suggestion of eating or food, all the staff encouraged me, and the mirrors constantly reflected my problem.

On a memorable occasion I saw a reflection in a shop window which looked familiar. I was very pleasantly surprised when I looked closer and recognized myself. I had become a different, slimmer shape.

The gymnasium took up all my mealtimes with Tony watching me carefully all the time. I told him the truth about my dieting and even, when we ate together, enjoyed the diet he had given me. I noticed that he always ate almost the same diet as he had given me.

On long runs, 10 miles or over, Tony ran with me. His plan was to lengthen my stride for economy of effort, and speed me up. This was not as simple as it sounded. It required absolute concentration and it was very easy to slip back. But after my first month at the gym, with improved breathing, controlled diet and a longer stride, plus some single-mindedness, I was able to demonstrate my progress to Randal who was back in England for a few days and had come down to see what I had been doing. We went for a 10 miler. There were bottles of water put out every 3 miles. I finished in ninety-three minutes, eleven minutes faster than ever before and a personal best!

The gymnasium soon became my sanctuary from food and temptation, a place so dedicated to health that hunger was left at the door. Gradually the gymnasium with the regime of exercises, weight training and diet, took the place of all other activities except my running. One day I said to Tony, the stranger who was now my trainer and becoming a very good friend, 'I feel I am in danger of becoming totally self-obsessed.'

'I hope so,' he said approvingly.

15 New Regime

My new regime demanded I step up my mileage from 25 miles to 50 miles a week.

Soon I was running the occasional 10 and 13 miler and was in the process of opening up new thresholds of personal endurance.

Diary

I came in from a 13-mile run, my calves screaming with pain and an icy chill paralysing the rest of my body. I asked Warwick to massage my legs, but I couldn't stand still long enough for him to do it. He put me on the bed, stripped off my tracksuit and rubbed my legs for a few minutes. I asked him to get me a drink and he disappeared to the kitchen and forgot all about me.

I was starkers on the bed, getting colder every moment and quite unable to move, even to get under the covers. I had made the mistake of trying to do this run with another person, a man, and we went too fast and did not stop for water breaks and my dehydration was clashing with my hypothermia and terminal exhaustion. It took me about an hour and some enormous effort to get up and walk to the bathroom and turn on the bath. With another colossal effort I got a drink of water. After the drink and I'd got into the hot bath I began to feel a little bit better. But the paralysing cold and the exhaustion stayed with me all day. After the bath I slept for two hours and then began to feel a little human again.

I told Tony what had happened and he suggested that I should always have a change of warm clothing and a high-protein drink prepared ready for my return. He is able to judge pretty accurately my precise capabilities and is always pushing me to the limit. The mistakes are usually self-inflicted, when I think I know better than he does and try to do a little bit too much.

Tony gave me a recipe for the high-protein drink which we called the Life Reviver.*

I was now firmly established on the 'Belinda's Diet Phase Two – lose 3 to 5 pounds a week'.

This diet was a salad mixture of carrots and apples, sultanas, pears, oranges, celery and yoghurt, three times a day. It alternated with a day of 'normal' low-calorie eating.

I was also eating a great deal of dried fruit, especially figs, dates and apricots. Dried fruit has much more sugar than fresh, but releases the sugar more slowly than, say, chocolate; psychologically, it is better to binge on dried figs than doughnuts or sweets and it does not encourage further erratic eating. Tony encouraged me to take Spirulina tablets three times a day as a protein supplement to help build up my new muscles through running and weight training.

My diet was going against the newly accepted wisdom which advocates low protein and high fibre. The latter is a good way to maintain your weight or lose gradually, but I was trying to lose a stone a month and could not afford to take on extra calories with the carbohydrates. In fact Dr Atkins in *Diet Revolution* stresses that a 'protein only' diet will result in weight loss because the body first burns up carbohydrates, then it turns to using fat for

* See p. 162 for recipe.

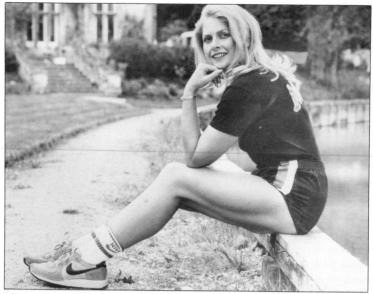

This was the picture which appeared in the *Daily Mail* and the *Sun*, and made me known internationally. After this my phone never stopped ringing. *Photograph: Associated Newspapers Group Ltd. Reproduced by kind permission.*

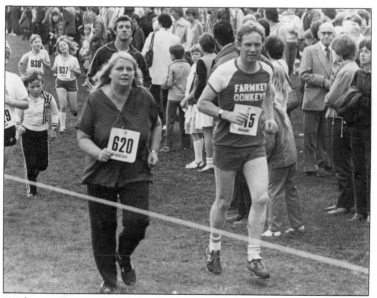

With my stepson Randal, who got me going towards the end of the nearly disastrous Banbury Fun Run. I weighed about 17 stone. *Photograph: Tudor Photography. Reproduced by kind permission.*

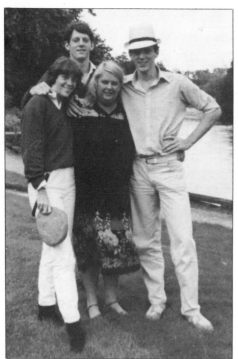

Left: With my three youngest stepchildren. From the left, Caroline, Alexander and Michael. *Photograph: Warwick Charlton.*

Below:Warwick, my husband, who helped me so much. I am weighing about 17 stone in this picture. *Photograph: Alex Charlton.*

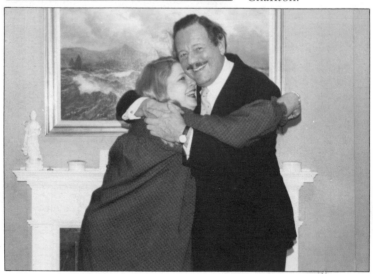

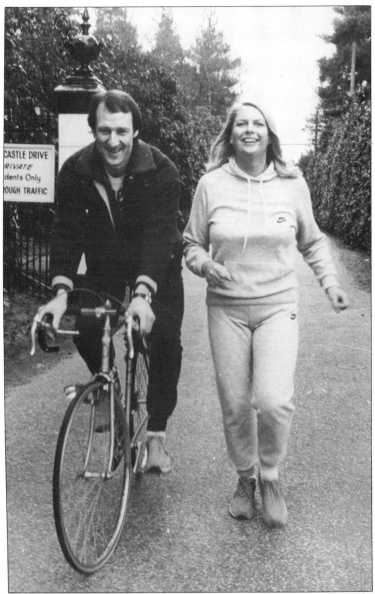

A training session with Tony Drinkwater. He ran with me and helped me weight-train. I am weighing about 13 stone in the picture. *Photograph: Simon N. Rowley. Reproduced by kind permission.*

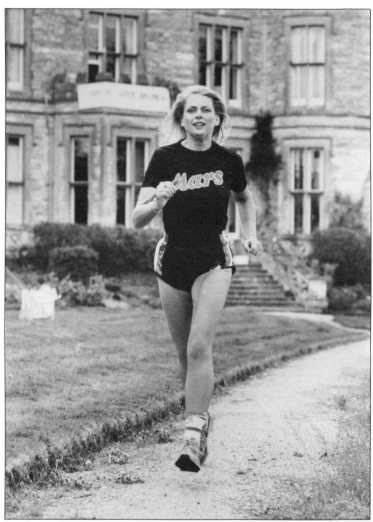

A week before my marathon. I'm worrying about my abcess, but trying a little run around the garden. *Photograph: Associated Newspapers Group Ltd. Reproduced by kind permission.*

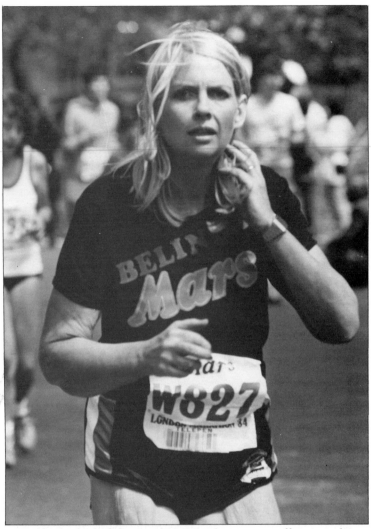

Towards the end of the London Marathon. I am suffering and not at all sure I will make it. *Photograph: Sun Newspapers. Reproduced by kind permission.*

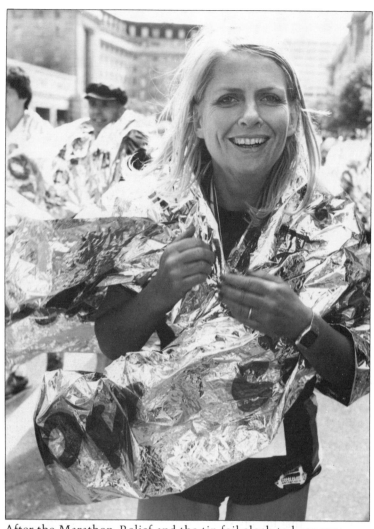

After the Marathon. Relief and the tin-foil cloak to keep me warm. *Photograph: Associated Newspapers Group Ltd. Reproduced by kind permission.*

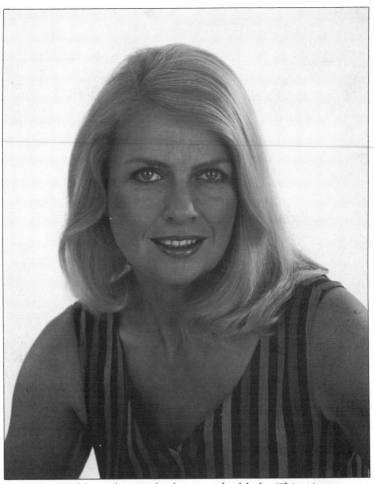

I became visible and a much photographed lady. This picture appeared in *Woman's Own,* one of the many magazines and newspapers that ran my story. *Photograph: Woman's Own. Reproduced by kind permission.*

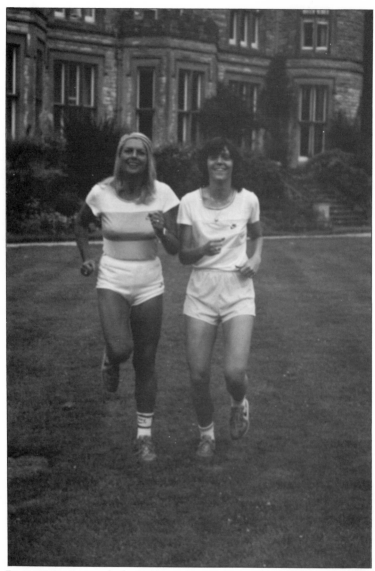

Because I run regularly I can eat twice as much as my nineteen-year-old stepdaughter Caroline without gaining weight. She and I are enjoying a gentle jog round the garden. *Photograph: Peter Stuart. Reproduced by kind permission.*

energy. As long as there are no carbohydrates in the body you can eat more calories than you burn up and still lose weight. Dr Atkins warns us though to be wary of fruit which has a high carbohydrate level. All the time I was losing weight I ate a great deal of fruit, so I must assume I was doing something right, but maybe I could have done better on less fruit.

I became very aware of energy levels in my body and would quickly eat an apple or banana if I felt my energy take a dive.

Actually, simple fresh ingredients, made doubly attractive by extreme hunger, can be a delight. An ordinary cottage-cheese salad can become delicious – adding fruit and nuts adds sweetness and texture. I must confess that my interest in gourmet food has waned a little. I can get quite turned-on by a flapjack or a particularly nice yoghurt.

When I first began training the gym mirrors constantly reminded me of how far I had to go. As an incentive there was always a slim young man in view effortlessly going through the routines, while I stumbled, puffed and suffered for three three-hour sessions a week. I found I tended to stick with exercises which made me look least repulsive. It was just as well that I could not see the ones that had me lying on my back and waving my legs in the air.

I found my weight training remarkably beneficial. It loosened up my upper body, and arms and shoulders moved more freely. My breathing also greatly improved. Flesh and flab was falling off my body, but not always in the right places. Tony told me that weight training would give me uplift for my bust, stomach and arms. And it did. The result is that I may not be as good as new, but I am a great deal better than I deserve to be and can now stand naked in front of the bathroom mirror and not cringe.

Diary

I am now running 50 miles a week and doing strenuous work-outs in the Olympian Studio three afternoons a week. The work-outs are non-stop against the clock for one hour each, and then a rest and repeat. The weight is falling off – but do I deserve it! Tony and I are constantly experimenting on how to fuel me with the minimum of food for the effort extended. We get it right most of the time, but with so much fatigue I sometimes find the effort of eating difficult, particularly as I cannot eat for two hours before a work-out and I don't want to eat after a run. So I sometimes under-eat (a thing I never thought I could ever do) and then fall to pieces and don't sleep and start sticking straws in my hair.

The weight lifting and exercises have done wonders in tightening up my body. When I first went to the gym I said it would take a crane to lift my breasts and I was planning plastic surgery, but Tony claimed that with weight training and some skin-therapy treatment from his wife, surgery would not be necessary. He even said I would not need a bra by the time he'd finished with me. I thought this improbable, but there already has been the most amazing improvement.

Every morning I crunched a potassium pill to replace the salts and minerals lost through sweat, a multivitamin pill, and two of my six daily Spirulina pills.

Tony places great value on Spirulina, these bright green strange-smelling pills, this source of concentrated protein. It has very little carbohydrate and a great many minerals, vitamins and amino acids; consequently, it is considered a good diet supplement.

I am not sure if it was effective or even necessary, but I did manage to build up my mileage to 50 a week and I did work out for at least nine hours a week as well as leading a busy life.

My diet was low in everything, so perhaps Spirulina was, as Tony affirmed, that little extra that made all the difference. Certainly I felt the new regime was working.

16 Because it's There

So long as my progress was followed on television every two weeks there was an added incentive to do well. But I was also aware of the price I had to pay for this vanity. My success would be publicly acclaimed, but any faltering on my part, any suspicion of faint-heart, would be publicly exposed. Sometimes, usually after a television show, failure seemed a remote possibility, like an accident that always happens to other people. But every now and then I was reminded that the settled serenities of life were being upset by accidents all the time.

A great Olympic athlete like Steve Ovett could not complete the 800 metres, was taken to hospital and the medical cause remains a mystery. Television gave a close-up of Ovett's agony and profound frustration. If it could happen to someone like Coe, or a world beater like Mary Decker, why not me?

Television made me feel like two people. Belinda on the air, an image without a physical body, was poised, confident and articulate. I felt, when on television, that I could not fail and it showed. But there was another person, the Belinda off the air and most unsure of herself; the one who crawled mewling out of bed every morning to run the cold deserted roads, gasping for air, groaning inwardly, longing for it all to end and to lie down and sleep for a year. There were the endless gym routines and the diet, which touched every moment of my day.

My other self, away from the television image, seemed to

concentrate entirely on herself: personal bests, pounds lost and gained, awareness of aches and pains. I felt guilty and sorry for my family, they must have felt ignored and deserted although they denied they felt neglected (especially my husband), and totally shared my enthusiasm.

I often asked myself – why do it? One classic answer, of course, was 'because it is there'. This is the reason mountaineers give – I was running the London Marathon simply because it was there to be run. Another real motivation was to change, to take control of my life, to make my living not just bearable but worthwhile. I was running for my life, I told myself and I should never forget it.

Of course I sometimes flirted with the idea of breaking out, of living normally, of going to London to an art gallery or theatre, but I could not risk breaking a routine now structured into my life. I visited friends and relatives as rarely as possible to avoid eating the wrong foods.

On one occasion I broke this rule to visit newly wed relations. I knew days of planning and hours of preparation would go into the welcoming meal. To make provision for this, I starved for two days so that I would be able to do justice to the feast. By the time dinner was served, I sat down in tummy-rumbling anticipation. Because of my diet, my meal had been specially adapted. I was served a minute piece of chicken breast, half a spoonful of peas and two small carrots. No sauce, no potatoes, no pudding.

In four mouthfuls my meal was eaten and it had not touched the sides. They had gone to tremendous trouble and a measure of self-denial to serve a meal suitable for me. But I was so disappointed I vowed never to eat out again or, if I did, to make sure I had a good supply of food with me. In fact I had started to carry around fresh apples, dried fruits and nuts. My husband called it my nosebag and it did look odd when produced in smart restaurants.

Dieting was always difficult for me and not many days went by when I did not cheat a little. But I was losing a regular 3 pounds a week, eating only fruit and vegetables, and fish every other day; but I did eat generous quantities made possible by the calories burned while running. I maintain now that, as long as I run between 30 and 40 miles a week, I can eat twice the amount eaten by my nineteen-year-old-step daughter without gaining weight.

For the first time in my life I felt really well, full of vitality and energy. I felt so good I could go off pop.

The work-outs in the gym firmed up my muscles and helped to burn up more fat. I used to be surprised at the people who congratulated me on the running. For me the real effort went into the weight loss. Compared to that the running was a doddle. The dieting so took over my mind that I had erotic dreams about food.

The gymnasium was the easiest place to contain my craving for food. Everyone there radiated control and self-discipline. Tony used to talk to me about the right foods I should eat. He made a salad sound exciting and a cream cake positively nauseating. He was constantly weighing me and encouraging me. He always advised me to eat enough and his obvious confidence in me made failure an impossibility.

Tony used to talk about me running 15 and 20 miles in a matter-of-fact way so that it seemed so attainable, but he never underestimated the effort or minimized the training required. What he did was remove the fear. At weekends he ran miles with me, increasing my pace, keeping me on track for my target. He gave up a great deal of his spare time to run long, cold wet miles with me to bolster my confidence. While I was on a diet, so was he. He described diet foods so that they would interest me. He talked about parsley bursting into flavour. I remember one day when I was uncharacteristically depressed by the sagging after-effects of my weight loss. He drove me to Christchurch where his wife Muriel ran their health and beauty clinic, Studio Olympus.

Muriel made me feel marvellous with a relaxing body massage to release my tight muscles and stimulate the blood flow. She then gave me faradic treatment with minute electrical impulses to stimulate the muscles and galvanic treatment, an electrical flow of current to aid the absorption of enzymes to help break down fatty tissues. She also offered sunbeds, facials and electrolysis, which I appreciated but reluctantly declined. The treatment had not only raised my sagging tissues, it had also raised my spirits as well.

My running was going well. I was tackling 8–10 mile runs confidently, clocking up 50 miles a week.

My biggest improvement had come with my speeds; I was determined not to be last in the Marathon. I was confident I could run 26 miles, but I was still innocent of many of the problems that beset the aspiring long-distance runner.

17 Bring on the Clowns

The Ferndown 10–mile run was my first public test and was covered by television. Tony and I practised round the route, twice round a 5–mile circuit.

On the day, hundreds of people lined the street route. This was my longest competitive run and thoughts of the Banbury Run made me uneasy. I was now better known and hoped there would be no collapse à la Banbury. At 12 stone I was looking better and my movements had begun to flow, to move more smoothly due to the weight training.

Before the start I did a radio interview and photographers took some pictures. I also showed off with stretching exercises as I had been taught, but with unnecessary enthusiasm. I set off on the run, feeling good but aware of a slight pain in my right calf.

Over the next 7 miles the pain became worse. Tony and my friend Valerie were running with me but they were absorbed with their own running; indeed, Valerie had an old leg injury troubling her. Eventually the pain was so bad that I had to concentrate just to place one foot in front of the other. I could hardly see where I was going. Other runners bobbed up and down in front of me in the distance, and I heard people cheering, but their shouts seemed to fade as I was taken up completely with the agony of my tendon. I had three miles to go and felt I had to stop. Valerie, running in front of me, was slowing down and in a lot of trouble. Tony had disappeared. I thought enviously that he was probably soaking in a bath drinking a cup of tea by now. In the event he was waiting anxiously at the finish with my tracksuit and refreshment.

What had started as an adventure was turning into a nightmare.

As I rounded a corner a fresh bellow went up from my husband, family and friends. 'Come on Belinda – you can do it!' Could I indeed? I doubted it. I struggled on to another corner, to be greeted with more encouragement. They saw I was wilting, that something was wrong. Valerie was still in front of me and I thought I could not go on. Then I saw the finish about 300 yards ahead. I picked up my feet as I had done in all those training sessions and overtook Valerie who, for months, had been pulling me along in training runs. I passed the finishing line in a best personal time of eighty-nine minutes for the 10 miles, ten minutes faster than I had run the distance before.

It was all over, or so I thought. In the excitement of finishing I had actually forgotten the pain in my calf, but it did not forget me. After a bath, food and rest, I felt a lot better and tried to stand up. A piercing pain stabbed through my leg, so I sat down again. I found I could not stand and I was only two weeks away from the training half-marathon Tony had insisted was my real test. It was to take place in Bracknell near my home town of Wokingham, in front of all my family and neighbours and it was to be televized.

The next day my leg was worse so I went to the doctor who said, 'You have strained your Achilles tendon. Complete rest for two or three weeks.'

I felt physically sick, I knew that it would never have happened if I had not shown off for the photographers before the run by doing fancy stretching exercises. It was my stupid vanity getting me into trouble again. Tony told me I had to do as the doctor advised: stop running.

A few days later my husband had a marvellous idea. Who had the most valuable legs in the area? Who knew better than anyone how to look after an athlete's legs? Answer: the physiotherapist for the leaders of the first division: the Southampton Football Team.

I asked TVS if they would help me meet with the team's manager who, in turn, recommended Don Taylor to treat me.

While Don gave me treatment TVS filmed. The team's manager Laurie MacMenemy told me not to be taken in by all the publicity. 'Remember,' he warned, 'the publicity won't run for you, you'll be running on your own, and they will all forget about you when its over.'

The physiotherapist, Don Taylor, gave me better news. 'With care your leg will be better in ten days.' All I could do was wait.

Without the running my spirits and willpower over food weakened. In one week I put on 3 pounds, as much as I had been losing with the running. My adrenalin was not flowing, everything seemed to be about to close in on me.

Not only did I have to be physically fit, my mind also had to be right.

Laurie MacMenemy's remark, that I was running on my own, stuck. But he is not quite right, I thought. My leg problems had been shown on television and recorded in the local newspapers; there was much speculation as to whether I would be able to run well enough for the Marathon.

I was deluged with phone calls, letters, postcards, all wishing me well, most of them from people I had never met.

Rosa Turner, who helped me in the house and had become involved with my project, said fiercely, 'I won't have it. None of us will. If you put on weight again, you will have to answer to me. I have told everyone you can do it, you can't let me down.'

Then there was my stepdaughter Caroline, who smilingly surrendered all her clothes to me when I eventually got down to her size 12. She also planted my water on the long runs and took over domestic duties while I was out running.

I used to sneak up early in the morning to her room while she was still sleepy and resistance was low. I used to select what I wanted from her wardrobe and ask if I could 'borrow' these things. A grunt was taken to be 'yes' and also a snore.

When I went into Ringwood or Bournemouth or Christchurch, people said how pleased they were I was up and about and hoped I would soon be well enough to run the Marathon. I would not exactly be running this marathon on my own – if their support meant anything.

My spirits were revived and I went back on my diet. I visited the gymnasium and went swimming. On the tenth day I tried out my injured leg. To my delight it held over a slow 5 miles. My weight had shot up but I was back in business again, off and running.

My next test was the half-marathon at Bracknell. This run highlighted one of the problems of the long-distance runner: how to judge precisely the correct amount of fluid to drink before or during a long race.

Running around the countryside on my own, there was always a handy bush if nature called. But in a large road race, with thousands lining the streets, it could be embarrassing. In most Fun Runs they have portable toilets at the start but never enough. In large marathons they also have toilets along the route.

In Bracknell the queue for the loo was so long that I did not bother. Then the gun went for the start of the race, and I immediately wished I had taken the trouble to go before. I also remembered that the television cameras would be on me for most of the race. This was to be a long race in more ways than one. I finished the 13 miles in extra-fast time, knocking about ten minutes off my personal best, but my spur was not to get the smart bronze medal they gave me but to find a loo and fast!

This is a not uncommon problem. With an organized Fun Run you are given water every three miles, and this is where the problem lies. On training runs you are not always used to taking on so much water and you have to be careful not to drink too much before you start.

Tony was very pleased with my performance in the half-marathon, particularly with the faster times and no sign of tendon trouble.

Meanwhile my old invisibility had given way to national media coverage of my story so that everywhere I went people recognized me, treated me like an old friend.

My family reminded me not to get too big-headed – which I was. Caroline named me 'Superstar' and had a T-shirt made for me with 'Superstar' printed on one side and a pair of old trainers on the other. Whenever I showed television videos of myself I was 'superstarred' by a family determined to keep my feet on the ground.

The runs were even longer now and I still felt very reluctant to climb out of bed and train in grey light on a wet early morning. Once out, as ever, my senses came alive after the first gruesome ten minutes. I smelt the sweet warm rain and the scents of the trees and bushes, the wind whirling around my arms and legs. Spring was emerging, tiny leaves, sticky buds, crocus and snowdrops and the crisp, clear sunshine. I remembered the days when I could hardly lumber up the hill a few yards; when it was an effort to walk downstairs and climb into a motor car; when all I saw were the insides of shops and restaurants and my home.

I had become such a familiar figure in the countryside that even the squirrels seemed to accept me. The dogs no longer came rushing out to chase me off. I was now one of them, just part of the early morning scene. Passing the wood I looked out for my rabbit, a large old gentleman with one floppy ear, who would slowly and rather grandly lope alongside me for a few yards before sitting down for a rest.

He was one of my regulars! And so were the drivers who passed me every morning, who always waved or flashed their lights. The little pony in the field used to trot up to the fence and whinny. I loved and felt part of the familiar landscape around me: the tiny trees, self-seeded and struggling through the undergrowth; the dozens of different shades of green and gold and the soft springy peat underfoot with the bright green tendrils of fern peeping through. This was a Spring I would always remember.

I had been lucky. I remembered some of the letters I had received from the people who seemed so alone and who battled without help, without the recognition of television, the spur of a loving family and friends. There were so many people with terrible illnesses and weight problems, with no one to turn to.

People began to speak as though the Marathon was just a formality. There was talk of a book, more television programmes, personal appearances and lectures. Magazines were ordering articles on running and diet and, after the British press, there were orders from European and American publishers.

But running remained my absolute priority. I was trying desperately to shake off a final stone in weight as Tony had insisted before the Marathon on 13 May. He thought my best running weight was 10 stone, and was determined I should get there.

I loved the attention I was getting but sometimes my nerves were stretched as I tried to keep up with the writing, television appearances and the running. One day my husband asked me how I was, and I threw a stepladder at him. The stepladder missed, so I threw a bowl of coleslaw as well. This time I hit my target and burst into tears, but felt better. Warwick looked confused, he also looked quite funny with coleslaw running down his face and my tears turned into laughter. Fortunately he also saw the funny side, but insisted I ate some of the coleslaw before he forgave me.

18 Second Opinion

Three weeks before the Marathon my health, which had been brilliant apart from tendon trouble, let me down. An abscess developed on my back at the base of the spine and was so painful I had to stop running. I hoped I had enough energy in my 'energy bank' to get me through. Four days later I began to worry about losing my ability to run.

Warwick was the first to sense my restlessness and warned me against trying to run.

'Your body is in superb condition,' he said. 'If you accept the medical advice from both Tony and the doctor, you won't run until the Marathon. I think the break will do you good.' I knew he always looks searchingly at me for signs of strain and had recently remarked on the danger signals of tetchiness and dark rings under my eyes. I knew that I had stopped running far too early before the Marathon. Ideally you should stop three days before, not three weeks. I announced I was going for a little run. Warwick tried to stop me.

'Have you talked to Tony?'

'No.'

'The doctor?'

'No.'

'Then you had better make an appointment.'

He began dialling the number but I was out of the door and away before he could get through. I did not want to see the family doctor; he had looked after me when I was seriously ill and, although he approved of reasonable dieting and exercise, he thought the Marathon was excessive showing-off and would not give his approval. He had previously suggested that I get a second opinion, which seemed reasonable, and I went to a cardiologist. He turned out to be a 'born again' jogger who ran marathons himself. He gave me absolute approval despite a slight heart murmur. My own doctor accepted the cardiologist's approval but he still did not think this marathon running should be encouraged.

My doctor prescribed antibiotics for the abscess and said that it might be better in time for the Marathon, it was difficult to say. It depended on whether the antibiotics were able to do the trick. They did not. A week later and the abscess was no better. My doctor sensed my rising panic and prescribed some even stronger antibiotics. Still no improvement. By now my doctor responded to my desperation and began hitting me with everything he'd got, but he warned me that there was no instant cure. I was not satisfied. It was painful just walking and the Marathon was only a few days away. I would try magic if necessary. Then my stepson Michael, the medical student, came for a weekend visit. I showed him my abscess.

'You need that lanced,' he said. 'Try to get somebody to do it.' This seemed like positive advice. At least it was something different and I was desperate.

I got a cab and went to the casualty out-patients in Poole. The sister in charge flatly stated that I did not classify as an emergency. 'Why didn't I go to my local doctor?' Well, I could see him in the morning, but I was running a marathon in five days' time and I was desperate. The sister was not moved.

'You are taking up valuable time,' she said. 'There are people here who really are emergencies.'

I was not so easily put off. I began grovelling. I would do anything. I had become convinced that this treatment was the only way I would be able to run the Marathon.

Finally, and grudgingly, she relented. 'As you have come so far and you are in pain, you might as well see the doctor, but I cannot promise treatment.'

The duty doctor was a young woman who did not look much older than my stepdaughter Caroline. I had struck pure gold. She examined me straightaway, she understood perfectly. Yes, she would lance the abscess. She had followed my progress on television and thought I had courage. 'And you are going to need some,' she added. 'Because this is going to hurt a lot.'

It did, and I think the young doctor suffered as much as I did. We both seemed to have tears rolling down our faces.

'I'm sorry I can't do more,' she said, 'but you should be over the worst. It's just a question of building up your strength. Good luck in the Marathon.'

After that I regarded Michael as a medical genius. My recovery was dramatic, the lancing effective, no doubt the antibiotics also worked, and I felt I had done everything I could.

Three days before the Marathon and I felt fitter. I also started eating under the direction of Tony, my trainer, and Randal by mail and telephone. They and all the books agreed that it was time to start carbo-loading, to eat carbohydrates which would give me plenty of quick energy. I was given the go-ahead to eat pasta and potatoes, rice and bread, plus a few cakes and biscuits and chocolates.

It was over six months since I had eaten cakes and biscuits. I had rather hoped that I had lost my taste for sweet things. To my delight and dismay they tasted absolutely wonderful. The first thing I ate was a shortbread biscuit. Sheer nectar I thought. Then a slice of fruit cake – I could not believe anything tasted so good. Up to now (apart from the odd, highly secret chocolate) the closest I had come to anything sweet was some natural yoghurt with a few raisins. Then I had some chocolate, a packet of chocolate Minstrels; I could not believe that there was anything as good as that! I loved the taste and the feel of them. I found the chocolate buttons comforting to have in my pocket and I could feel the bag in my hand with the smooth round Minstrels ready for crunching.

I ate a hot sausage roll and remembered the unfamiliar greasy taste and decided I did not like it one bit. I had lost my taste for meat and fat, but sweet things were a joy.

I ate a flapjack with caramel icing. Heaven. I had fantasy dreams about toasted tea-cakes, scones and cream and jam. All these were delights which, as a serious eater, I had previously considered to be too frivolous for my attention. I tried eating some more meat, the first in six months. The spaghetti Bolognaise tasted fine, but I thought I would have preferred it with a cheese sauce instead of meat.

The next day after my first carbo-loading, my stomach was upset. Randal and Tony had both warned me not to overdo it. According to my training instructions I could put on as much as half a stone in weight before the Marathon to give me plenty of available energy to burn up. I expected to lose half a stone during the run, but meanwhile it was 'snout in the trough' time with a clear conscience.

I ate ice cream with chocolate sauce – a dream. I ate a chocolate Florentine cake with fruit and nuts. Food for the Gods. My body and appetite were screaming out for sweet sticky cakes and biscuits. Once I had started it seemed impossible to stop. To hell with the steak and chips, all I wanted now was sponge cake, gateaux, macaroons and chocolate cake with ice cream. I knew I would have no trouble at all in putting on half a stone, but what would happen afterwards? Would I be able to stop? Could I ever again be enthusiastic, even with Tony's prompting, over fruit-and-vegetable salad, grilled cod and spinach? Compared with chocolate cake and Minstrels, my high-fibre, non-sweetened breakfast cereal was very unappealing. My hidden box of secret After Eight Mints had not prepared me for this deluge of delight. I was carbo-loading and enjoying every minute of it.

There was another final delight in store for me before the Marathon and it came from Television South. They told me they were going to film a pre-race Special at my home. They were going to show the film the day before the race.

The format for the pre-race show was a party in my garden for all the people who had supported me. I made some vague noises to Vic Wakeling and Mark Sharman that I was interrupting my final training schedule, but as I loved television it was probably the nicest thing that could have happened to me.

The day they filmed the party was bright and sunny. I was bundled off at first light to the hairdresser and facial experts. Professional make-up experts were something I liked very much. In a half hour they filled in all the cracks and took ten years off my age or so I imagined. They certainly reinforced my confidence. At this point some people, mostly my family, thought my confidence was quite high enough, as it was. A few more television booster shots and it would be in orbit. Naturally I disagreed, but I had to admit that I was more than compensating for all those years of social invisibility.

I was fortunate to live in a very picturesque Gothic castle by the River Avon. The grounds were large and elegant and TVS set up a marquee, tables and chairs. Champagne corks popped, the gardens were full of smiling people. Hanging across one of the turrets was a large banner saying: 'Good luck Belinda'. I absorbed the scene and identified the faces: Tony, looking very different in a lounge suit; my patrons at the Olympian Studio, Don and Mary Howard; my stepdaughter Rachel Anderson who had come down with some friends, the Southend Joggers. I had converted Rachel to jogging. She had taped my television programmes and showed them to her friends, and they had decided to follow my programme. Subsequently, they had competed honorably in 5- and 6-mile races.

Rachel told me how fit they felt and how much better they looked and how much weight they had lost. She also told me I was a folk heroine.

'Marvellous,' I thought. 'They'll be composing songs about me soon to sing round the camp fires: "Belinda of the hungry mouth, is the fastest slimmer in the south!"' It was a novel experience to be a role model, to have your views sought by young women who, in the past, would probably not have noticed me. I had to be careful about what I said. The days of shouting to make myself heard were over.

Even my sister Susan was listening to me, probably for the first time in her life. 'How did you do it?' she asked, not troubling to hide her admiration. It was a lovely situation with a big sister who had always had the upper hand since childhood. I did not recall her seeking my advice before. Not only that, she handed over all the smart clothes she had grown out of which now fitted me, but she added the proviso that, if she lost weight following my programme, she might be wanting them back.

As I took in the scene of the television party and the guests raising their glasses to toast me, I felt more than a twinge of guilt. The only person I had done anything for so far, was myself, and I was also the one whose self-indulgence had so nearly brought me down in the first place. I was really having my cake and eating it. It was all there: beautiful setting, food, champagne, friends, relations and neighbours and Vic Wakeling, Mark Sharman, Bob Evans, Gareth and Domic – the team from Television South. I was tempted to try the champagne but, with only a day to go before the Marathon, I did not. Anyway I felt high enough as it was.

The climax of a lovely day came at the end of the party when a magnificent cake, in the shape of two running shoes decorated with yellow sugar roses, was brought in. Cake was in line with my carbo-loading training schedule so, although I refused the champagne, I spent most of that evening eating cake. I had never really liked the rich fruit birthday cake before, but did I enjoy this! It was the most delicious and exotic thing I'd ever tasted.

During the party a photographer from the *Daily Mail* came to take my photograph. The next day the *Daily Mail* carried a double-page spread of me sitting in the garden by the river in running shorts. Overnight my story went national, and then even international. The following day the *Sun* also ran a double-page spread and then the story ripples spread. The phone went berserk. I was offered two film parts, both pornographic! I was asked to do photographic modelling, some of it respectable; I had to laugh at the demand for my body which had never been thought of very highly before. If anyone had looked at me a year ago, the response would have been a shudder.

There were offers to appear on television, write magazine articles, make personal appearances, open things and endorse products. I even got some passionate love letters from fans, and now everybody was recognizing me in the street. I was a popular newsworthy package and I was loving every minute of it.

When I asked Warwick what I should do about the demand for my new image by the media, he said, 'Stand up and enjoy it.' I think he had never been so proud of anything before in his life.

19 Night Before

It was the night before the Marathon and I was having difficulty getting to sleep.

There was a quiet, almost tentative, knock on the door of my bedroom at the Farmers' Club in Whitehall, London, just past midnight.

'Belinda, it's me.'

I lay absolutely still, eyes closed. Warwick had taken a separate room at the Club so that I would be sure of a night's rest before the race. We had gone out to an early celebration dinner at my favourite Italian restaurant for a traditional pre-race spaghetti. It was the San Marino, near Hyde Park Gate, and there the large family party gathered. There were my seven stepchildren: Randal, Victoria, Rachel, Thea, Alex, Michael and Caroline with their respective spouses or partners. My mother, Kathleen Chapman, and my two sisters, Susan and Jo, were there, as well as assorted cousins and friends. I appreciated the warmth of their support, their festive mood and their absolute confidence that I would complete the course, but I desperately needed to wind down, to rest. They understood and I left the dinner party early on my own to return to the Farmers' Club at 9 o'clock. Warwick had booked us in and I was touched to find a note from him to say that there were separate bedrooms so as not to disturb me when he returned from the celebration dinner. But I was not surprised when I heard the tap on the door and Warwick calling my name.

I knew he, too, wanted reassurance.

I had been spinning off on my own, further and further away from him. I was either training or dealing with the media, almost always with other people.

The Marathon was a big day for him too; it had become as much a part of his life as of mine. I lay in the dark waiting for him to stop calling my name and trying the door. I reasoned that I would be better off on my own, with a small chance of some sleep, than with my husband and no chance.

Earlier in the day we had driven round the course, from Greenwich docks to Woolwich Ferry, along the Thames, past the historic windjammer, the *Cutty Sark*, and the Isle of Dogs, through Rotherhithe and Wapping docks, back round the Isle of Dogs again, down Wapping High Street to the City of London, Blackfriars, Victoria Embankment, the Palace of Westminster and the Mall. The finish of the 26-mile-385-yard-race was the other side of Westminster Bridge.

I went round the course in my mind, my thoughts straying to the television and radio interviews I had to give before and after the race.

My appointment diary was solid for the next three weeks. I was used to pressure, that of a large family and work, but not the increasing demands on my attention and time as a new celebrity.

I tried desperately to sleep, to crawl into a corner of my mind and sleep. But my mind was spinning. I concentrated on the run and decided that it would be a release from pressure. There was nothing else I should be doing that day. So long as I completed the course I could not go wrong. I had nearly reached my goal. But I was not alone. There would be 20,000 other people running, over 3,000 of them women, experiencing a similar mixture of excitement and apprehension. I would soon be one of an exclusive worldwide club: a marathon runner. There would never be anything again like my 'first-time marathon'. I weighed 10 stone 5 pounds. I had aimed to be 10 stone.

When I woke it was 5.30 in the morning and there were dark circles under my eyes. My mouth was dry and my legs stiff. God, I thought, why *am* I doing this? Maybe I could stay in bed and say I had overslept. I could roll over and forget all about it, I would not be missed in the crowd.

I put on my heated rollers, bathed and made up my face. I did not often bath, make-up and curl my hair before a run, but this was different; I was determined to look my personal best. I had put out my clothes the night before and checked them a dozen times. The firm-hold athletic bra, the cotton pants (not too tight), clean Nike socks, white towelling shorts, cotton shirt, Nike Pegasus running shoes, grey tracksuit, running number W827 with four safety pins, headband and maroon waterproof tracksuit to go over the lot. A jar of vaseline to stop chaffing, a towel, brush and comb and make-up. Plus a £5 note and some change for the phone, the latter in case I had to drop out and make my own way home.

I dressed ceremoniously, a ritual. I told myself that I was a Japanese warrior preparing for hara-kiri. I faced a full-length mirror, stood to attention, saluted and marched out of the room. I felt a bit light-headed, there was no strain just a rather unreal feeling like a dream. I drank just one cup of tea and ate nothing. I never ate before a run. I was careful not to drink too much.

I picked up my bag and strolled out of the Farmers' Club to Whitehall and the empty London streets. It was 7 a.m. and dawn was breaking over Nelson's column as I walked through Trafalgar Square to Charing Cross Station to board one of the Marathon trains laid on by British Rail to take us to the start at Greenwich. I already had my ticket.

The station was alive with runners: men and women, all ages, shapes and sizes, chattered compulsively, drank tea and coffee from plastic cups. One man had travelled down from Scotland and another from Los Angeles. One woman kissed her baby goodbye as though for the last time. All the ashtrays were empty.

People talked about their coffee and tea drinking like drinkers in a bar. 'Let me see, I've had three, no four – daren't have another.'

Our train number (previously allocated) was called. This prompted nervous adjustments to underclothes and shoe laces. We shuffled off to take our seats. I sat back trying to appear nonchalant, reading a *Sunday Times*. For a few moments there was silence in the carriage, then someone spoke and the spell was broken.

One person had just developed a bad cold, another had left a family crisis. Someone else had a car breakdown, and a small wiry man of sixty said he had missed the bus and had to hitch. Wherever everybody lived, the biggest concern had been to get to Charing Cross Station in time to catch the Marathon train for Greenwich. We runners had been advised not to drive to the race start, the road would be closed to traffic we had been told.

Someone said, 'All we have to do now is run the race – the difficult part is over.' He meant the training and the waiting.

I was worried I had not had enough sleep until I spoke to other competitors. Many had not slept at all, no one more than five hours. Some confessed they had not had a good night's sleep for over a week.

When the conversation inevitably turned to training I discovered that, in a carriage of ten people, possibly a cross-section of competitors, I had probably done more training than most. For me it had become a grand passion and taken two years. Latterly I was running 50 to 60 miles a week, while most people in my carriage were satisfied with an average of 30 miles a week.

Someone asked if I had any foot, leg or other injuries and found they had inadvertently pressed the conversational jackpot button. My pulled tendon and abscess stories were played back in full.

At Greenwich station I was grabbed off the train by BBC 'Grandstand' reporters. I felt I was too hyped up for the race, too nervous to give a good interview. I just could not think straight but, when I saw a playback later, I seemed reasonably calm and articulate.

In the park, at Greenwich, there was a mighty array: 20,000 competitors talking, drinking, standing, sitting and lying on the grass. I felt diminished for a moment by the vastness of the crowd and then felt a surge of gratitude that I was part of it. There was the smell of embrocation as muscles were rubbed and others shared a pot of vaseline. That prompted me to get out my pot and to smear an especially vulnerable place under my bra straps.

Queues to the portable lavatories grew longer, there was not much else to do except some stretching exercises and survey the more eccentric participants. One man was dressed as an emu. He told me he had almost collapsed in a previous marathon when it rained and made the feathers exceedingly heavy. Another man, dressed as a waiter, was running with a tray and a bottle of mineral water. A team from Norway in Viking dress planned to run in a replica long boat. Some were dressed as clowns and others as panto dames, one was a convict with a ball and chain, another was a baby in a nappy. One elderly male competitor had a heavy money belt filled with coins for charity. I thought that, before the race was over, he might regret the extra weight, to say nothing of the noisy jingling.

I thought many of these competitors were foolhardy, the Marathon was difficult enough without a costume handicap. But Christopher Brasher, the originator of the London Marathon, himself a world-class athlete, thought the clowns, the Viking long-boat runners and other eccentrics part of the fun, the carnival, that was an essential ingredient of the London Marathon.

The runners, the people of London and the millions watching on television shared a great day, the spectacle of men and women extending themselves to the limit, mostly for the sheer joy of living. There was also some pain and anguish. All of us were showing off, too, and that, as any child knows, is very satisfying.

I overheard some talk about the dreaded 'wall' we were supposed to hit at about 20 miles, the moment when the body's supply of glycogen, the energy source stored in the muscles, was spent, and the body was forced to switch to stored fat for fuel. The feeling would come suddenly and without warning. One moment you could be running normally, the next moment you would feel as though you had literally run into a wall, reportedly a harrowing experience. I am not sure if I experienced the 'wall' in training. I did have some difficulties. Maybe, I thought, I will run up against it for the first time today.

I knew many people running in the Marathon but, as I looked around the park, I did not see one of them. I began to feel very much on my own. Then, to my amazement, I saw Tony striding towards me. He had driven since dawn from his home in Hampshire to reach me before the start. It was an incredible achievement to have found me amongst 20,000 people, one I took to be a good omen.

Tony smiled and swung me round, he too was caught in the excitement of the race.

'You will do well, I know it,' he said. 'I am your bag man. Here to carry your vitamin pills, recovery fruit drinks and warm clothing for the end of the run.

'Remember, Belinda, run slowly at first, pace yourself. Do not go too fast, too soon. Time each mile with your stop-watch.'

I had a final relaxing massage before going to the starting area.

20 The Marathon

The start was split into two sections: Red at one end of the park for fast, experienced runners, some of whom would be competing in the next Olympics and the rest of us at the Blue start. The road to the starting line was split up by posts giving different times. You estimated the time you hoped to take and stood in the appropriate section. This way you would not hold up the faster runners or be swept along in the fast stream.

I chose to stand by the four-hours-thirty-minute post, but was secretly hoping to run in four hours fifteen minutes. I wondered of my abscess would give me any trouble. I gave Tony my tracksuit as an icy wind whipped up, bringing goosepimples to my now trembling limbs. He gave me a black dustbin liner to wear and discard after I had warmed up. A final good-luck hug and Tony disappeared and I was on my own.

The sound of the starting gun was the signal for us all to surge forward and stop. Twenty thousand bodies are a lot of people to get moving in one direction at the same time. After precisely seven minutes of shuffling we were at last away, running.

My aches and pains and misgivings were forgotten. I had never felt so good. I wanted to kick up my heels and sprint, but I knew this was wrong. The atmosphere embraced us. Thousands of people lined the streets. It was exhilarating.

I knew the long route through London stretched before me, but all I could see was an avenue of friendly faces.

I was running in the 'Mars' livery (red, gold and chocolate brown) like a chocolate Mars bar. A man trotted past me and said, 'Hello, the girl from Mars – I wouldn't half like a nibble of you.' The crude joke made me laugh, I relaxed and felt delighted to be running.

Most spectators and runners recognized me from television and I was cheered by name as though I was the only person running. At each corner they shouted, 'Come on Belinda!' or, in the East End, 'Go on gal – you can do it!'

In the East End the streets were dressed with bunting, there was a pub-party atmosphere! They watched from deck chairs and tables with great pots of tea and cans of beer. People were hanging out of windows and decanted from the pubs. A policeman wearing a red false nose made me laugh so much I nearly fell. Musical spectators played us on and others rigged up stereos and radios to provide background music. The effect was one of joyous festivities, a pure delight to be part of a ritual, we the competitors pushing ourselves through the pain barrier, they, the spectators, urging us to greater sacrifice.

The first 13 miles was surprisingly smooth. Part of the time I ran alongside the crew representing the Viking boat; they planned to run together throughout the race. No easy thing to do when everyone has a different pace. About halfway they disintegrated, as a boat, but all of them finished.

As I settled down I began to feel I was the only one running. 'Belinda, come on Belinda,' they chanted, lifting and carrying me along the early miles faster than I intended. All the hours, days, months of training were paying off, the adrenalin charging through my body as the sun shone and a brisk wind blew my hair around. On some corners we were greeted by a blast from a brass band. There must have been a dozen bands en route and, as the notes from one faded, they were taken up by another.

Round the docks euphoria gave way to grim reality, the smooth tarmac to cobblestones and we stepped up and down kerbs. At 18 miles I began to feel threatened for the first time.

Over half way and only 8 miles to go, but the end seemed a very long way off. At 20 miles I had been running for over three hours. At this rate, I thought, I should finish within my anticipated time of four hours fifteen minutes.

Then the crowds started to thin out, the cheers faded and exhaustion began to take over. Now all I could hear was the sound of my own breathing, the feel of my feet hitting the road. I believed I had been running for as long as I could remember and was doomed to run the streets of London forever.

The 22-mile mark was agony. I got paralysing cramps in my stomach, my legs became lead weights, my head throbbed and I wanted to die.

I gave up stopping at the water stations because my legs buckled as I changed pace. If I went down no amount of willpower would get me on my legs again.

As I ran I saw many casualties by the roadside, runners lying with bleeding feet, faces distorted with pain and exhaustion. One man had hit the 'wall' and was running as stiff as a board, only helpers kept him upright. A girl sat on the kerb rocking backwards and forwards, tears streaming down her face. In her I saw what might happen to me. A television interviewer put his arm round my shoulder and leaned on me. I tried to shake him off.

'How do you feel Belinda?' he said. 'How do you feel?'

I could not believe he was serious. I felt it would be difficult to finish if he held on to me any longer. I was angry and then I remembered how much I owed to the media, how they had encouraged me. I curbed my anger and talked to him as I ran about the crippling cramps in my stomach and legs that felt like ton weights; aching head and muscles, the overwhelming desire to crawl into a corner and die and, most of all, the doubt that even now, after twenty-two miles, I was not sure I could finish.

I was totally preoccupied with staying upright. Running over

London Bridge alongside the Thames and Victoria Embankment, I passed St Paul's Cathedral and Cleopatra's Needle.

My thoughts were of putting one foot in front of the other. I saw my family waving as I turned into the Mall, but I was too exhausted to lift my hand in acknowledgement and hoped they would understand. I tried a smile. I felt nothing in the world existed but the road just in front of me and the pain in my stomach. Getting there... Near the Houses of Parliament I heard people cheering again, 'Belinda, Belinda, Belinda!', saw Westminster Bridge and knew I only had to cross the bridge. But what a very long bridge it is. Suddenly people clutched me, told me to stop. I ignored them, I knew I must not stop. Then I came to. People dressed in Mars uniforms supported me.

'It's all right dear,' they said, 'you can stop now, you have made it.'

I turned around and saw, for the first time, the big Seiko finishing line behind me. I had run the London Marathon.

A microphone was pushed in front of me. I do not remember what I said. Press photographers took pictures of me. I was drawn to one side by reporters, and then towards even more reporters. Then TVS took over.

Throughout the run I had seen their familiar faces; they wrapped a foil cloak round me for warmth. What I needed was liquid, a drink of anything. I asked the television crew to get me a drink. They asked me how I felt. I was swaying, having trouble standing upright, but more words and pictures were required. I was led off to get my medal and a free Mars bar, but still no drink, no sign of a place to rest and recover.

I followed the film crew to the Jubilee Gardens, the meeting place for runners, solid with hundreds of people. Some women were sitting on a bench with their shopping bags and they made room for me to sit down. I was grateful to be off my feet, less likely to collapse.

The television team had finished their job but felt they could not go off and leave me alone; then Tony appeared and set to work. He gave me a drink and put me, limb by limb, into my tracksuit. He gave me things to eat. Almost immediately I began to feel better, happy it was over.

We walked slowly back over Westminster Bridge, my body stiff and awkward from the sitting. Now I enjoyed every second. People smiled at me, patted me on the back, congratulated me by name. At that moment, on that day, I was probably the most visible person in London.

21 New Body Takes Over

It was the happiest moment of my life. I had run the London Marathon in four hours thirty-two minutes on the official recorded time. By my stop-watch it was four hours twenty-five minutes – it had taken me seven minutes to get to the start line after the gun had gone off.

If I thought my telephone was busy before, it was nothing compared to what happened now. Eventually I had to leave it off the hook for a few minutes' respite.

In shedding half my weight I had also lost a good fifteen years of age and could comfortably mix with my own age group again. Now I could lead a sizzling new life. When people asked me how I felt weighing in at 22 stone plus, I felt I was talking about another person. Could it really have been me? That woman whose only exercise was walking round a supermarket? Who used to sit in the car to prepare herself for the ordeal of climbing a few stairs or walking a few yards? Who had the energy to bathe, or walk round the shops but not both? Who dreaded parties or meeting people because it also involved looking in a mirror and not liking the reflection?

I was at home in my new body. The question now was how my family would accept the new personality in the new body. I had nothing to fear. They accepted with absolute love and delight. My daughter Caroline resigned herself to the fact that none of her clothes were her own any longer. She protested mildly about my pinching socks, but that was the one sign of revolt.

My weaknesses are still there, not far beneath the burnished new surface. I yearn for all the fattening foods, sweets, cakes, biscuits and comfort snacks.

I promised, after the Marathon, to make up for the neglect I inflicted on my family during training, and I try to do so. I still stay relatively clear of the kitchen and go on fruit fasts for a few days if my weight is up a few pounds.

My sex life has improved. My husband finds my new slim shape much more interesting, and I enjoy the attention I receive from other men. When I walk into a crowded room I am no longer socially invisible. Not only am I slim, but my skin, eyes, hair, poise and overall figure have improved.

It seems strange that running and dieting makes your hair glossy, puts a sparkle in your eye, but it does. Your manner is relaxed and confident. You no longer think, as I used to do, that no one values your opinion.

With clothes, as with more serious subjects, I listen to what other people have to say, but in the end make my own decision. This is new for me and rather daring. The temptation is to wear clothes as tight as possible to show off my new shape, to be dashing and different, to try every colour because I imprisoned myself so long in dark blues and blacks. I had to decide on my new look. Sporty or sophisticated? Was I going for glamour or tasteful elegance? Dress as a mature woman, or a young woman? I settled for a sporty look, with a touch of glamour for the evenings.

I rarely have to carry a suitcase anywhere. Where were these gallant gentlemen when I was fat and needed them? I am often offered lifts, now I don't mind walking. I can cross my legs and fold my arms and fit into any sized chair.

My dry-cleaning bills are right down because I do not have so much out front to catch all stains or crumbs. Because I am recognized I am also smarter. Even an outing to a local shop is preceded by careful grooming. I do less food shopping, take fewer taxis and buses. The money I save on food and fares goes on cosmetics, facials and hairdresser.

My stepchildren are proud of me and do not mind kissing me in public. I can actually hug someone again. Everyone seems willing, including my elder sister, to take my advice on dieting.

I am invited to parties and functions specifically, and not just as an appendage to my husband. My body bends and moves more gracefully and is now almost as good as it was fifteen years ago.

I know I could not have lost the weight without the running and could not have run the Marathon without losing weight. Now that the weight is off, I know I can keep it off as long as I run regularly and eat sensibly.

I must finish this adventure, as I began, on the subject of food.

If I eat normally, which I find difficult, I would not gain weight. When I want to lose weight, I cut down on food and increase my running. So long as I run I know I will feel well and be able to cope with everything.

I believe a diet is only good if it suits the individual. A diet only works if you can stick to it. On a long haul, such as mine, it is probably better to switch around, to bring variety to a tedious business.

There are basically three types of diet:
1. high in protein and fat,
2. high in carbohydrates and fibre,
3. low in calories and fat.

They all work in different ways. I lost my weight with a mixture combining the best of these diets. I evolved my own diet, which broke down into three phases:

Phase One: Belinda's lose a-pound-a-week diet is basically low calorie.

Phase Two:	Belinda's lose three-pounds-a-week diet is high in protein and low in fat and carbohydrates.
Phase Three:	Belinda's maintenance diet is virtually vegetarian, high carbohydrate and high fibre.

I find this the most satisfying, the easiest to stay on. But to lose weight on it I am strict with myself and cut fat to the minimum.

Successful dieting is not so much what you put into your mouth, but what goes into your mind. You need to be relatively unworried, absolutely determined to face up to your weaknesses and to identify why you fail. Maybe you always pop into a bakers on the way to work to buy cakes? By changing your route you avoid temptation.

Break a set eating routine and establish a brand new one. Cut down on the number of places at home you associate with food. I found myself spending a great deal of time in the bathroom as the only room in the house in which I did not eat. If you eat in front of the television, turn it off and go out. If you cannot leave your family, take up a hobby which involves using your hands.

My biggest problem is eating while I type. Although I am using my hands, at the end of each sentence or paragraph I need a nibble, so the writing of this book is a struggle in more ways than one.

Sometimes in desperation I wear a tight pantee girdle and tight trousers so all the time I am working I am conscious of an uncomfortably tight midriff.

Once you have made up your mind to run yourself thin as I did, you will be pleasantly surprised at the support from family and friends. If you are a born fattie as I am, however, the way to maintain a healthy weight is to act, to eat carefully and run, run,

run. There is a certain amount of suffering involved, but to act is to suffer.

I know I will always have to make an effort to maintain my size 12 figure. Running began for me as a faint hope and became a grand passion. It is certainly exhilarating and, from time to time, a gateway to absolutely pure pleasure.

Part Two

1 Important Tips to Know before Starting the Diet

I can eat twice as much as my nineteen-year-old stepdaughter Caroline and not gain weight. I can binge on a big evening meal and then run it off in the morning, all I need to do is eat sensibly and run. If you follow my dieting and exercise plan you will be able to do the same.

We all know how to lose weight. Eat less, eat differently, eat only what you really need. I can add 'eat for the enjoyment of eating'.

Through running and exercise I have been able to speed up my metabolic rate which means my body burns up energy faster. I use more calories and can therefore eat more calories.

So efficient was my body at storing fat, that my medical stepson Michael said, 'You should be grateful. Come the famine you would be one of the last to die.' It was cold comfort to me weighing 22 stone and with ambitions to run the London Marathon. But in two years, not only did I lose 11 stone in weight but I built up my stamina and metabolic rate by running.

Get Set

Set yourself a date to start dieting, not too far off but not so immediate as to trigger a panic reaction. Give yourself time to get used to the idea but not to forget about it. A week away is about right.

Prepare yourself as much as possible. Buy in the right food. At each meal tell yourself there are only so many more meals before the diet begins. Try on some clothes the size you plan to be.

Try not to think of the weight loss as a whole, but take it one day at a time. Plan to weigh yourself with witnesses. Meet up with some friends and relations at the same time each week and weigh yourself in front of them; their job is to tell you how well you have done. Write your weight on a chart and put it on the wall, then forget about it until the next week. Now you only have to diet for just seven more days to the next 'weigh-in'.

Break up your week with special activities to keep you away from food: swimming, aerobics, sport or a visit to the hairdresser. Go to the cinema (this can be dangerous ground because of the popcorn and sweets) or an art gallery or bowling alley. Enrol in night school and take up a new hobby. I tried pottery. Have you ever tried eating with clay-covered hands? Recognize and avoid eating temptations.

One of my favourite diversions was a visit to the Roman Rooms at my local Recreation Centre in Ringwood. It is difficult to eat in a sauna (the food would go soggy), or lying on a sunbed or while you are being massaged.

Family Help

I bought and prepared only food that was on my diet. If my family wanted anything different they were happy to get it themselves, and gave me prior warning so I could avoid the smell of their cooking or the sight of their eating. I would hide away in my bedroom with my cassette player.

Try ready prepared and frozen meals if you do have to cook for a family. They reduce the time spent in the kitchen preparing food. If you ask your family for help, you may be surprised at how co-operative they can be.

Divide Your Day

Divide your day into four non-eating sections with a goal to aim for in each section. 8 a.m. to 12 noon/ 12 noon to 4 p.m./ 4p.m. to 8p.m./ and 8p.m. to midnight or bedtime. Reward yourself for good behaviour with a cup of coffee in a coffee bar, or an apple or a walk in the woods, or a soak in the bath.

When desperate, try some exercises, these will kill or suppress hunger pangs.

Plan the day hour by hour. Identify time when you are at food risk. Feed your family first and clear away. Then concentrate on your own meal and do not be tempted to eat as much as them. Delay eating for as long as possible. I find that the later in the day I start to eat, the less I eat.

Fill every minute with positive non-eating activity.

Goals

Set weekly goals with a ritual weekly weigh-in. Lose 2 pounds by Monday and 2 stone by Christmas. Choose a firm date as your long-term goal, a birthday or anniversary or the day you plan to get pregnant, but keep to it.

When you reach your goal congratulate yourself on the weight loss and straightway go for another goal. Remember, a non-realistic goal will put you off dieting forever. Always aim for what is possible.

Some people may tell you that you have lost enough weight, often the person closest to you. Do not be conned. Rely on your mirror, your scales and your commonsense before discarding your diet.

Your Enemies

Refined sugar is enemy number one and is probably the most difficult to avoid. It is hidden in a great many basic foods such as bread and 'unsweetened' cereal.

Boredom and anxiety are enemy number two. Fill every minute of your day. Idle hands will pop food into waiting mouths. Running and physical exercise does wonders to relieve stress, anxiety and tension.

Breaking your routine is your third enemy. This makes you vulnerable. You may be doing very well, then you visit a friend or guests arrive. There is a crisis at home or at work and your routine of running and diet becomes unimportant. If you do break your diet or miss a run, do not waste a moment in handwringing. It does not matter if you stumble and fall as long as you get back up and continue running and dieting.

It is harder to gain weight than to lose it. Cheating for two days does not necessarily mean you will gain but, if you diet for two days, you may lose a pound or two. It is never, ever, too late to start again. Each time you stumble you do have to recover the mental approach and the resolve that started you off.

Here, as a guide, are the World Health Organization's recommended figures for daily energy intake from food, for the average person.

Age	Calories Men (11st)	Calories Women (8st 8lb)
16–19	3600	2400
20–29	3200	2300
30–39	3100	2200
40–49	3000	2200
50–59	2800	2000
60–69	2500	1800
70+	2200	1600

This reflects a general slowing down as we get older, though if you are still doing a great deal of exercise in middle age you still require a good many calories. Elderly, energetic farmers, for example, have been observed to require as much as 4000 to 5000 calories. I am in my mid-thirties and, when running 30 to 40 miles a week, I can eat 4000 calories a day.

I guarantee that, if you follow any of the three eating plans combined with running, you will reach your goal weight. *But you must see your doctor before you start and tell him exactly what you plan to do.*

Sugar – the Empty Calorie

I tried to cut out refined sugar and fat during the five-month run-up to the Marathon when I was losing over a stone a month. I cut down on carbohydrates as well.

In the Western world we now manage to eat less but at the same time become fatter. The main cause is refined sugar, often hidden in what we eat, and lack of exercise.

In their 1983 report on obesity, the Royal College of Physicians stated categorically: 'Sugar is an unnecessary source of energy in a community with such a widespread problem of overweight.' The report went on to say that 'Sugar is not only without value, but deprives the body of vitamins and minerals we would otherwise obtain in healthy food. Sugar is an empty calorie which supplies nothing but energy.'

Sugar can even become addictive. Eat one bar of chocolate and you will want another. Refined sugar overwhelms the body's natural reaction to unrefined sugar in fruit or starch in vegetables and cereals.

Eating refined sugar causes an artificially high blood-sugar level and then, because of the body's defence system, artificially lowers the blood-sugar level which, in turn, recreates the craving for sugar.

129

It is now accepted that refined sugar is a contributory factor to heart disease, diabetes and diseases associated with the digestive tracts, including cancer.

But how do we know when we are eating refined sugar? Many 'unsweetened' cereals contain a lot of sugar. Cornflakes and All Bran are both culprits. In order to help I have included some foods to beware of:

Foods High in Refined Sugar

	Percentages
Sugar (white and brown)	100
Peppermints	100
Meringues	95.5
Boiled sweets	85.9
Drinking chocolate (dry)	73.8
Golden Syrup	73.8
Toffees	70.0
Jam	69.0
Mars Bars	63.8
Ribena (undiluted)	61.0
Chocolate (plain)	59.5
Chocolate (milk)	57.0
Sugar Puffs	56.0
Bounty Bar	53.6
Bournvita (dry)	52.0
Horlicks (dry)	49.4
Fruit cake	46.6
Wafers (filled)	44.5
Chocolate biscuits	43.4
Ginger nuts	35.7
Jam or treacle tart	33.5
Branston Pickle	32.6
Rusks (for babies)	30.5

Sponge cake	30.5
Muesli (packaged)	26.2
Tomato ketchup	22.5
Fruit salad (canned)	22.5
Ice cream	22.0
Rich tea biscuits	22.0
Malt loaf	18.6
Fruit yoghurt	17.9
Doughnuts	16.0
All Bran	15.0
Jelly (water)	14.2
Currant buns	14.0
Salad cream	13.4
Coca-Cola	10.5
Rice Krispies	9.0
Canned sweetcorn	9.0
Lucozade	9.0
Cornflakes	7.4
Energen crispbread	7.4
Peanut butter	6.7
Tomato soup (condensed)	5.6
Orange and lemon (diluted)	5.6
Weetabix	5.6
Baked beans	5.2

Foods high in refined sugar are unnecessary.

The body, however, does need sugar in a natural form. Dried fruits are higher in natural sugar than fresh fruits. Bananas, grapes, mangos, cherries and pineapple are higher in sugar than other fruits. Onions and beetroot are also high in natural sugar. Stay away from high sugar fruits if possible. Concentrate on melons, grapefruit, apricots, raspberries, plums, oranges, tangerines, blackcurrants, strawberries and blackberries.

For really rapid weight loss here is a list of foods very low in sugar.

Foods Low in Sugar

	Percentages
Natural yoghurt	4.5
Fresh milk (skimmed)	4.5
Leeks (boiled)	4.5
Almonds	4.2
Carrots (boiled)	4.2
Coconut	3.7
Loganberries	3.5
Peas (canned)	3.5
Crispbread Ryvita	3.1
Tomato juice	3.1
Lemons	3.1
Peanuts	3.0
Gooseberries	2.8
Aubergines	2.8
Tomatoes	2.5
Parsnips (boiled)	2.5
Vegetable soup	2.5
Water biscuits	2.3
White cabbage	2.2
Wholewheat bread	2.0
Peas (fresh)	1.7
Cucumbers	1.8
Brussels sprouts	1.5
Puffed Wheat	1.5
Butterbeans	1.5
Runner beans	1.0
Lettuce	1.0
Marrow	1.0

Spinach	1.2
Celery	1.2
Cauliflower	0.7
Lentils	0.7
Spaghetti and most kinds of pasta	0.7
Potatoes	0.6
Watercress	0.6
Shredded Wheat	0.4
Rice	Trace
Porridge	Trace
Mushrooms	0.0
Meat and fish	0.0
Marmite	0.0

Fats

As well as refined sugar, I cut down on fats a great deal throughout my two-year running and slimming campaign, particularly during the last six months.

Doctors and nutritionists accept that saturated fat clogs up the arteries, creates heart problems and is dangerous in excess. It is the butter on the bread that causes obesity, and then the jam full of refined sugar on the butter on the bread. The bread itself is relatively innocent (although it does contain sugar); potatoes are even better. Again they are fine on their own but add butter and sour cream and cheese and then the calories and the problems start.

Exit Red Meat

I cut out all red meat and ate only a very little chicken or turkey. In a month I had lost my taste for red meat entirely – but I wish I could say the same thing for cakes and sweets. Red meat is full of saturated fat which threatens your health, as are all animal foods which contain a lot of saturated fat: meat, butter, lard, cream etc. Vegetable fats and oils contain polyunsaturated fats which are less likely to increase blood cholesterol.

All fats are fattening, however, so when you are cutting down, start with the saturated fats, then cut out the vegetable oils. The following shows the source of fat in the average British diet:

27%	from meat products
13%	from whole milk
13%	from margarine
13%	from cooking oils, lard etc.
12%	from butter
6%	from biscuits, cakes and pastries (these also contain refined sugar)
5%	from cheese and cream
3%	from eggs
9%	from other foods.

Give up red meat but make sure you get enough protein from low-fat sources. These are white fish, cottage cheese, eggs (the fat is in the yolk), low-fat cream cheese, lentils, peas, beans and other pulses. (Remember, canned baked beans are quite high in refined sugar.)

I have studied many diets and many methods including those of Weight Watchers, Geoffrey Cannon's *Dieting Makes You Fat*, Dr Atkin's *Diet Revolution*, Audrey Eyton's *F Plan Diet*, the Beverly Hills diet, and advice from athletic experts. There is something to be learned from all of them especially, in my view, from Geoffrey Cannon because he, like me, strongly advises running as a permanent solution to a weight problem. He also agrees with me that a crash diet has little or no permanent value.

I have tried many diets during the past twenty years, but never more intensively than during my two-year Marathon build-up, when I lost 11 stone and achieved a weekly mileage of 50 miles.

2 Two-Part Diet

My dieting was basically in two parts. The first eighteen months was done quite slowly with lots of lapses. By the time I had lost 6 stone and was down to 14 stone, I had got thoroughly fed up with the whole business but was feeling a lot fitter and happier, could fit into a size 18 dress and would probably have left it at that.

The second phase of my diet was much more intense with the goal of the Marathon coming increasingly closer. I changed into top gear and lost weight at a steady 3–5 pounds a week for five months, while building up to run 60 miles a week. The high degree of energy output certainly helped my weight loss, probably by as much as a pound a week. Nevertheless, you do not have to run a lot to lose weight on my diet.

I have raised my metabolic rate through running and exercise but, nevertheless, have a very low pulse rate (40, resting), and naturally low metabolic rate. Those with a higher normal rate (60/80) will lose weight fast on my diet. The higher your metabolic rate the more calories you burn and the quicker your weight loss.

Delay Eating

Many nutritionists suggest you start with a good breakfast to give you energy and stop hunger pangs later on. Accepted thought has begun to change on this and I agree that appetite is not just stimulated by hunger. Other factors are involved. You only need to smell something good to eat and your body craves for it whether you have just eaten or not.

A place is often associated with eating; walk into a restaurant and you will immediately feel hungry. Eating itself stimulates a desire to eat more, so I try to eat only when I am really hungry, or I feel my energy level dropping, or I am suffering a temptation due to an eating stimulus.

I find that the later in the day I start to eat, the better it is. Every time I want to eat I ask myself if I am really hungry, or is it just an outside stimulus? Usually I am not really hungry.

If I give breakfast a miss, I can often last until 11 p.m. at night. That means less time for temptation once I have started eating. But be warned, it takes very little time for people like us to consume a great deal of food. Even if you don't eat until midnight, you can still eat a day's food in an hour.

An advantage of eating a lot at night means that you are less likely to feel hungry in the morning.

Get Confident

Set your mind right to feel confident. If you feel you will succeed then you will succeed. Treat any lapse as a temporary slip-up and not a mortal sin. Real foodaholics, and I am one, have to put as much mental effort into losing weight as they do into passing examinations, obtaining degrees, bringing up children, doing a job or becoming good at their sport.

Ask yourself 'Why am I overweight? Is it one reason or several?' Overweight is not necessarily the result of greediness or laziness. There are many other reasons. Sometimes a fat person's body is just too efficient at storing fat. Under stress we will comfort ourselves by eating. Other people may take up drinking, gambling or lose their temper. Whatever prompts us to eat too much we are quietly and considerately inflicting retribution on ourselves only.

First, we have to decide on our method of dealing with stress, tension and worries. They must no longer continue to spoil our lives. It is in this determination that we must be very selfish. We must not allow any outside influence to interfere with the diet and exercise regime we decide to follow.

Friendly Co-operation

We must ask our family and friends to co-operate with us. There is a price. They will not get the same attention and the meals cooked for them.

Instead, they will share in our good intentions and our diet, and enjoy good food which will make them feel a lot better. If they do not like this they will have to get their own meals. Remember, this is not a forever diet, but I hope, like me, it will change your eating habits permanently. You can continue to enjoy normal high-fibre, low-fat, low-sugar food and never really have to diet again.

High Fibre

A few words about fibre. It is important you eat sufficient fibre. The less time food hangs around in your body, the less likely it will add to your weight problems. Fibre is also very filling and satisfying, but passes through the body at a healthy rate.

Medical opinion agrees that food high in fibre causes less problems due to bowel infections and reduces the risk of cancer of the bowel.

Here is where most fibre is found in the British diet:

48%	from vegetables
30%	from cereals and bread
12%	from nuts
10%	from fruit.

Foods High in Dietary Fibre

	Percentages
Bran	44
Bran cereals	27
Dried kidney beans	25
Haricot beans	25
Dried apricots	24
Desiccated coconut	23.5
Energen bran crispbread	20
Dried figs	18.5
Dried peas	17
Dried prunes	13.4
Lentils	11
Wholewheat pasta	10.0
Brazil nuts	9
Wholemeal bread	8.5
Peanuts	7.6
Oatmeal	7.0
Sultanas/raisins	7.0
Baked potato	2.5

Naturally, you are able to eat more potato than, say, bran, and so consume a higher degree of fibre. A normal helping of bran may be $\frac{1}{4}$ ounce on your cereal.

This would represent 3.1 grams of fibre in one serving. A baked potato, however, eaten with skin would weigh around 7 ounces and represent 5 grams of fibre in a serving. (Instant potatoes (1 ounce with water) represent 4.7 grams of fibre.)

As long as you eat some foods in these categories you are

getting sufficient fibre.

Phase Two: Speed-Up Time

On Belinda's 1-pound-a-week diet, I managed, with many lapses, to lose 6 stone. I got down to 14 stone and a size 18. I felt wonderful and went on holiday to Israel where I lay in the sun and ate for one month. Although I was a long way from my goal, I felt as though I had done it and was dangerously close to stopping altogether.

Fortunately, my acceptance for the Marathon was waiting on my return. The Marathon plus the television prompted me to start again and lose 5 stone in five months.

This diet does not allow for human frailty. You have to stick to it and do running. You must keep yourself occupied with non-eating activities. Spend time at the sauna, gymnasium and solarium, swimming, aerobics but, above all, run.

Structure your days as I did, with highlights that have nothing to do with food: a clothes shopping expedition, a visit to an art gallery, theatre, cinema. Play tennis or rugby or visit a sports show.

Get away from food and stay there. I made a rule always to travel with my nosebag so I would not have to go near snack bars or restaurants. I would always carry three or four apples, some grapes, a couple of bananas, figs, dried apricots and sometimes unsalted nuts.

Never buy food on a journey. Make your nosebag do.

First Eighteen Months

Weigh yourself on good bathroom scales, preferably digital scales which do not fluctuate. Invite a friend or relation to witness your weight. Write it on a chart and stick it on the wall.

Then forget about it until the same time, same place next week.

You can join a slimming club and weigh in every week. Weight loss is often uneven, some weeks you may not lose weight at all. Another week you drop between 5–9 pounds. So do not lose heart so long as you maintain a healthy average over a month.

Here is my guide for the gradual weight loss. Belinda's 1-pound-a-week diet

In General
Drink as much tea and coffee as you like. Use decaffeinated coffee to allow you to sleep and stop that jittery feeling caused by caffeine. Use skimmed milk and no sugar (sweeteners if you have to).

Eat as much fruit as you like, but remember that an apple is the equivalent to a spoonful of sugar in calories. Eat fruit but don't gorge on it.

Try not to eat too many dried fruits as they are very high in sugar but they do travel well. Never be caught short; although dried fruits have a high sugar content they are much better to eat than a bar of chocolate. Not only does the odd bar of chocolate spoil your diet, it is likely to trigger off an eating binge. If you stick to fruit and nuts this will not happen.

Always be prepared. Get into the habit of buying fruit nearly every day.

Another fail-safe is yoghurt. A bowl of natural yoghurt eaten slowly, with perhaps a few raisins and some bran, is very satisfying and so much better than a slice of cake.

The Diet

Breakfast
2 ounces unsweetened cereal: Shredded Wheat, Natural muesli,

All Bran, Bran Buds or Bran Flakes, or boiled or poached egg on slice of wholemeal toast with scraping of margarine, or 5 fluid ounces of natural yoghurt with six raisins, two chopped apricots, sprinkling of bran and All Bran.

Eat as much fruit as you like but watch the grapes and bananas as they are very high in sugar.

Lunch
6 ounces cottage cheese *or*
two eggs *or*
6 ounces tuna fish in brine or grilled white fish
Large mixed salad
Two slices wholemeal bread and margarine
1 dessertspoon slimline salad cream
Fruit
Yoghurt with raisins or natural maple syrup *or*
Chopped prunes and apricots or fresh fruit.

Dinner
6 ounces of grilled or roast poultry *or*
8 ounces of grilled or baked white fish
Sauce made with skimmed milk (parsley, Bearnaise, Hollandaise etc.)
4 ounces of jacket potato or boiled potato or rice
Peas, carrots, green vegetables
One serving ice cream or fruit sorbet or cream caramel
Fruit
Diet soda drink

Fruit or natural yoghurt as snacks when necessary, not more than 10 ounces of natural yoghurt or three pieces of extra fruit a day.

This basic diet can be varied of course, using as many green vegetables and spices as possible. Some vegetables should be restricted and not eaten more than three times a week. They are:

Beetroot	Mange-tout peas
Sweetcorn	Parsnips
Broad beans	Peas
Waterchestnuts	Baked beans.

Potatoes should be limited to one 4–ounce serving per day; rice to one 4–ounce (cooked weight) serving per day.

With the exception of avocados, which should be avoided, all other vegetables can be eaten in as much quantity as preferred.

All milk should be skimmed.

All yoghurt should be natural low fat.

As little added fats as possible.

No added sugar (use sweetener if necessary).

No ready-prepared meals.

All food should be freshly prepared and cooked as lightly as possible to preserve vitamins and minerals.

No red meat.

No sweets, cakes, pastry, puddings except for one treat a day: 2 ounces of ice cream, or two biscuits, or one scone and butter, or one toasted tea-cake, or one portion of jelly, or one glass of wine or spirit, or one teaspoon of jam, honey or chocolate sauce, or one ounce of cheese or single cream.

Demon Drink

Although I allowed myself one glass of wine a day, I would often save that up and drink seven glasses of wine in a day or two, perhaps on a Saturday night out. This is fine for some people but not for me; the alcohol would often weaken my resolve and leave me with a hangover which made me reluctant to run. It is best to try to cut out alcohol altogether. The drink will often lead to another drink and then on to some bad eating: the after-effects can cause a depression which is against everything I am preaching. If you are used to drinking, however, it is a mistake to give up too much all at once. This will lead to failure. Try to cut down gradually and, unless you feel you can really keep it under control, try to cut it out altogether.

If you feel you need a drink at a social gathering to boost your confidence, overcome nerves, or not to seem left out, a brisk run will have the same effect and you can always sip slimline tonic water. If you don't believe me, just try it.

Where There's Smoke

If you are a heavy smoker, I suggest you do not try to give it up completely while you are trying to lose weight. As with the drinking, if you attempt too much you are doomed to failure and will get nowhere. If running is part of your programme, however, you will find that you progress with running better if you smoke less.

I used to smoke usually when I was drinking. The moment I cut out drinking I found I cut down on smoking considerably. It is possible to run and diet quite satisfactorily while both smoking and drinking, but you will not do as well, or feel as good, as doing without.

I was running long distances while still smoking, but I discovered that an evening spent over a few drinks with perhaps five or ten cigarettes could put my training back a whole week. I found that even two or three cigarettes in an evening has a noticeable effect. Your legs may be going well but your breathing is being left behind.

Drinker's Bonus

The damage done by drink is not so noticeable. You can do

surprisingly well, while feeling like death, but a lot of drinking will slow you down and lessen your enjoyment of running. Most of all it greatly reduces your desire to go out and run and could well stop you running altogether.

There is a bonus though. Running is the only really effective cure for a hangover. I used to judge the level of my indulgences the night before by the distance I ran in the morning to get rid of the hangover. A 2–mile run was, say, a half bottle of wine, a five miler a bottle and a half, and 10 miler two bottles or more and a bucketful of remorse.

Housebound Eating Alternatives

If I could not get out, I organized jobs in the house or office to keep me away from the kitchen and food.

I work from home so it is very easy for me to find myself standing at the open door of the fridge looking for a little 'something' to nibble. Sometimes it was so automatic I didn't realize I was doing it. I then made a conscious effort to do something else. If I wanted a break from work, I would plan to water the plants, or sew on a button, or make a cup of coffee, or iron a shirt, or tint my hair, make a phone call, read the paper. I would always save something up to fill my break.

To avoid eating during the evening, I am told that gardening is very good on summer evenings, or embroidery or painting the bedroom.

Belinda's 3-Pound-a-Week Diet

Basically I would eat proper food only on alternate days. The days I did not eat I would eat only fruit or vegetables in restricted quantities. I drank as much decaffeinated coffee with skimmed milk and sweetener as I wanted. I did not drink alcohol. Every day I took a multivitamin tablet, a potassium tablet to replace the salts and minerals lost in running and six spirulina tablets. Spirulina is, as I explained earlier, a form of algae or scum found on alkaline lakes in Mexico, very high in protein and minerals and vitamins but totally non-fattening. Spirulina can be bought at most health-food shops. I stayed very healthy on this diet.

The Diet

Monday (non-eating day)

Breakfast
2 spirulina, 1 multivitamin and 1 potassium pills. Small bowl fruit salad, using grapefruit, orange, lemon and apple.

Lunch
2 spirulina
½ melon, small bowl of fresh fruit salad
Coffee

Dinner
2 spirulina
½ melon, small bowl of fresh fruit salad

(Sometimes I would eat more fruit than allowed, but I always stuck with fruit.)

Tuesday (eating day)

Breakfast
2 spirulina, 1 multivitamin, 1 potassium pills.
Bowl low-sugar, high-fibre cereal (All Bran, natural muesli, Shredded Wheat) and a few raisins, or
Bowl of natural yoghurt with raisins, 2 dried apricots, bran, a few nuts.

Lunch
2 spirulina
3 ounces of cottage cheese and green salad (lettuce, cucumber, celery, green pepper)
Fruit: banana and apple

Tea
Fruit: grapes, apple and orange

Dinner
2 spirulina
Six ounces grilled white fish
Boiled green vegetables (cabbage, spinach, sprouts, runner beans, cauliflower, broccoli) or
Green salad
Fruit

Wednesday (non-eating day)

Throughout the day I would eat:
6 spirulina, 1 multivitamin, 1 potassium pills.
Three portions of yoghurt, fruit-and-vegetable salad composed of:
12 ounces yoghurt
2 medium-sized carrots
2 apples

3 sticks of celery or endive or chicory
Small handful of raisins
¼ cucumber unpeeled
Small green pepper
1 pear
1 orange.

Chop up all the ingredients in the morning. Shake them well together in a container and divide into three equal portions. When ready to eat a portion pour 4 ounces of natural yoghurt, flavoured with a little lemon juice, over the salad.

My coach at the Olympian Studio, in Bournemouth, Tony Drinkwater, gave me this recipe and also recommended the Spirulina pills. He claims that he and his wife Muriel have used this diet with great effect at both the Olympian Studio and at their health clinic, Studio Olympus, in Christchurch. He told me that it acted as a diuretic to help flush impurities from the body.

Tony suggested that I had this salad once a week, but I found it so palatable and satisfying that I used to have it more often, usually on days I was at home and not travelling around.

It is important to buy the best fruit and vegetables and to buy daily to ensure they are as fresh as possible. You will be spending a great deal less on food for yourself, so you may as well get the best.

Thursday (eating day)

Breakfast
2 spirulina, 1 multivitamin, 1 potassium pills.
5 ounces natural yoghurt with raisins, apricots, high-fibre cereal, and bran *or*
Poached egg on toast with scraping of butter *or*
2 ounces of low-sugar, high-fibre cereal with skimmed milk and raisins

Lunch
2 spirulina
4 ounces tuna fish canned in brine
Mixed salad or coleslaw
Fruit

Dinner
2 spirulina
6 ounces of poultry
Green vegetables *or*
Salad
Fruit

Friday (non-eating day)
As an alternative to fruit you may eat only vegetables.

Breakfast
2 spirulina, 1 multivitamin, 1 potassium pills
½ glass vegetable juice
2 grilled tomatoes
1 slice wholewheat bread

Lunch
2 spirulina
Cabbage or spinach, cauliflower, broccoli – boil and flavour with
garlic and lemon juice

Dinner
2 spirulina
Green salad – lettuce, cucumber, celery, watercress, green
peppers, onion

Saturday (eating day)

Breakfast
2 spirulina, 1 multivitamin, 1 potassium pills
1 poached egg on toast *or*
Cereal *or*
Yoghurt
Fruit

Lunch
2 spirulina
5 ounces haddock with green vegetables
Fruit

Dinner
2 spirulina
3 ounces low-fat cream cheese and mixed salad
Fruit

Sunday (non eating)
Often I would be travelling on a Sunday and would take the fruit with me.

Breakfast
2 spirulina, 1 multivitamin, 1 potassium pills
1 apple, 3 dried apricots

Lunch
2 spirulina
1 banana, 1 apple, 4 dried figs

Dinner
2 spirulina
1 pear, 4 ounces of grapes, 3 dried dates

If you have extra fruit, like I did, only eat when you are severely tempted. Sometimes I would not eat until late evening, as almost all eating triggers off further eating with me.

It is probably better not to try elaborate recipes at this stage as this is a relatively short-term diet. Stick to white fish and cottage cheese as much as possible. Cut out red meat, fats, sugar, bread, potatoes, most root vegetables other than carrots, and anything pre-prepared. Stick to leafy green vegetables with the occasional portion of peas, sweetcorn or beetroot.

After the first three or four days, you are likely to feel as I did, a little light-headed and droopy with a foul-tasting mouth and lacking in energy. Your body will also smell unpleasant. Do not be alarmed. These are the toxins leaving the body. In a little while you will feel wonderful.

By the sixth or seventh day there is a transformation! Energy is restored and a feeling of well-being and happiness combines to make you feel on top of the world. You will also have lost weight. Depending on how overweight you are it could be as much as 10 pounds in the first week.

You may find you pass water more frequently and, because of the drastic change in diet and the iron in the multivitamin pills, you may need a mild laxative. This will all sort itself out eventually.

After the Weight Loss – What Next?

If I continue to run regularly I will probably never need to diet again as long as I live. If I am sensible about it, I can eat more or less what I like without gaining weight. This includes coping with serious lapses. When this happens I compensate with a strict fast for three days, eating only an orange and two apples a day. A short, sharp shock, gets my body on the right tracks again, and then I launch into my 3-pound-a-week diet again. In a week I feel happier and healthier and, in a very short time, maybe no more than two weeks, I can have lost half a stone or more and be slimline again.

I vow to stop the binge eating but recognize that there is a possibility that there will be a next time. This is the weakness I have to live with, but one which I will not allow to take over as I did before. I will not let myself gain more than 10 pounds in weight, before doing something about it.

I can maintain my weight with the following diet, as long as I run at least 20 miles a week and cycle about 15 miles a week. If I really stick to it and step up my mileage a bit, I can also lose weight.

Belinda's Maintenance Diet

Breakfast
5 ounces yoghurt, handful of All Bran, raisins, chopped apricots
Slice of wholemeal toast with butter and honey
Fruit

Lunch
7 ounces baked potato
6 ounces cottage cheese, mixed salad, coleslaw, beetroot
Fruit salad

Tea
Tea
Wholemeal bread and natural jam, butter
Cake, two biscuits

Dinner
Split-pea soup
6 ounces roast chicken, stuffing, 4 ounces boiled potatoes,

sprouts, carrots, gravy
Wholemeal apple pie and cream (small portion)

Snacks of fruit, dried figs, dates and one bar of chocolate a day.

This is quite a generous diet. The cakes and chocolate are there to try to stop the binge eating.

People who have been very overweight, like myself, do have an emotional problem with eating which is nothing to do with hunger. Five months after I ran the Marathon, I succumbed to a severe bout of comfort eating. I fell right back into my old bad ways, and put on 8 pounds in a month. I even found I could eat sweets while riding my bicycle, and I used to have a secret packet of chocolate buttons in my pocket all the time. I would eat a meal, then forage in the kitchen, open a tin of rice pudding, eat some leftovers and a whole packet of biscuits.

When this happened, I planned to start my diet again one week ahead, and spent a week working myself up to it. I fasted for three days, went back on my 3-pound-a-week diet and, within three weeks, was back in shape again and feeling wonderful.

I then added a few more goodies to my maintenance diet, like the chocolate and cake, which I try not to eat but do not feel too bad if I succumb.

Health and Strength

Running and the resulting fitness increases your resistance to common colds, aches and pains.

Since I took up running, I rarely catch a cold, have a glowing, clear complexion and feel clear-headed and capable. If I do have a cold it is very slight and rarely lasts more than twenty-four hours.

The difference between being non-fit and super-fit is to be aware of how very good it is to be alive. The simple truth is that you cannot look your best unless you are fit. It can change an average-looking woman into a beauty.

You will find your brain is quicker and more responsive, more able to accept new ideas. I believe that running makes you better looking, brighter and bolder.

You are not afraid when waking up in the morning, there is no quaking in fear at those little buff envelopes with threatening letters from credit-card companies or banks. Neither a new business venture or a dinner party for twenty can shake your confidence. It is a wonderful feeling knowing you can cope – and for that you can thank the diet and the running.

3 The Running

Running is the least harmful and the easiest exercise for fitness. You can adapt it to fit your various stages of fitness, you do not need anyone else or any special equipment. You do not need to run a marathon to become fit and healthy, but you do need a goal. I believe that if you can run 5 miles in fifty minutes you are a fit person and your life should change dramatically for the better.

Anyone who is more than 20 pounds overweight should see their doctor and ask his advice. Tell him you intend to start running, beginning slowly and building up to longer distances. Your first few training 'runs' will, in fact, be walks.

There are a hundred good excuses for not running half a mile, 5 miles or 10 miles on any particular day. I have thought of all of them. A sore ankle, a dodgy knee, visitors arriving, an early-morning appointment, children who cannot be left, incipient colds, a wet tracksuit and so on. It can be too dark or too wet, too windy or too hot. It can make you late for work or the children late for school. Maybe you haven't slept well, or you have a hangover, or your tracksuit's in the washing machine. Perhaps it is nice and warm in bed and you want another little cuddle, you'll snuggle up now and run later. Oh yes, I know all the excuses – I also know you will do more cuddling and snuggling when you are slimmer and fitter than ever before. One of the hardest things is to get out of bed, into the tracksuit and out of the door. Once this is accomplished you are halfway there.

There are times when you should not run: when you have an injury or you have a bad cold or flu. Do not be tempted to attempt too much, too soon. Run on grass or cross-country to minimize injuries. If you are very overweight as I was and covering long distances there is an added risk of sore knees, so it is particularly important for overweight runners to have a soft running surface. Remember, running is the most natural thing to do. Your body was designed to hunt for food and to escape from predators. You are not asking your body to do anything out of the ordinary, but to function efficiently as it has done for several thousand years.

When people hear that I have halved my weight and overcome ill-health by running a marathon, I hear a lot of reasons why they do not do it themselves. Here are the most common:

'I'd like to take up running but I don't think I could do it. I get out of breath running for a bus.'

This is the 'left it too late and too far gone' excuse. It is never too late and I am not asking you to catch a bus. Most people who start running, usually set off too fast. First walk, then trot as gently and slowly as you can. In the early days try to work comfortably within your capacity. You will know when it is time to really push yourself.

Ideally, you should always be able to carry on a conversation while you are running. This comes with practice. Running is natural but technique helps you make the most of your particular ability. A few yards and then a rest was all I could manage when I began. My first run came after one month of regular walking. I ran for as long as I could, thirty seconds, and covered about 150 yards; my lungs felt as though they were bursting and I was pouring with sweat.

'I would like to run, but I never have the time.'

But there is time for a few beers at lunchtime. Time for dinner, time for a favourite television programme, time for a concert or a movie. Time to go to the lavatory or have a hot bath. Time to read, to smoke, to talk. There must be time to make the most of your life.

Running is a way of doing that. It appeals to all types, not just the leisured few. Most often it is the very busy people, high-powered executives, very busy housewives with small children, people who are under a lot of pressure, who need to find relief from tension and stress in running.

Busy people who run, find they have time to get even busier. The running helps them cope with pressure. The question for them is not whether they can find the time to run, but can they afford the time not to. . . .

Fitting it in takes some planning. Early morning is best but lunchtime or the evening is also good. It is a wonderful feeling to run in the dark. The night seems as smooth as velvet. It is cool and fresh and silent. Without familiar landmarks you can feel you are flying. An early morning start before dawn can reward you with some amazing sunrises and a glimpse at a secret world most people miss.

I have seen mothers running, pushing a baby in a pram, office workers running to work. Some people run up and down the stairs in high-rise buildings.

'Running is a waste of time.'

You can use running time to work out problems and think through plans of action. The knottiest problem will unravel as you pound the pavement. The secret is to empty your mind, choose a subject you want to think about and gently mull it over; it is remarkable what can be achieved. I have composed difficult letters, an opening paragraph to an article, worked out menus and complex arrangements for guests and written shopping lists. As a journalist, I always get ideas for stories on the run. Now I take out a pad and pencil to jot down any inspiration. I keep the notebook in a plastic bag to keep out rain and sweat. I think I can do as much work on the hoof as I can sitting at my typewriter. Three years after I started running, I still have to whip myself to get up and go out. I still flirt with the idea of lying in bed. But, fortunately for me, the running usually wins because I feel *so* good afterwards.

'Running is boring.'

You may prefer tennis or squash or Rugby, but how often do you actually get a game? All you need for running is yourself and your running shoes. You compete against yourself, beat your best time. Run through streets or the ever-changing countryside. Experience different sights and sounds every time you go out.

Run against or with a partner. Vary your run: a short route and a long route, a fartlek (a mixture of very fast and slow running), interval running (two minutes fast, two minutes slow for thirty minutes) and hill work.

'I am too old and too fat to run.'

Check with your doctor first and take it easy. No one is ever too old or too fat (well almost no one) to run.

I weighed 20 stone plus when I started at thirty-five years old. A friend of mine is a sixty-eight-year-old man who is 5 stone overweight. He took it easily and a year later is running 3 miles a day and losing weight without dieting. He has never felt better.

'Running is lonely. I have no one to run with.'

Once you start, you can join a running club and I guarantee you will meet people who are only too happy to run with you. Although it is more pleasant to run with someone else, it can become an excuse, in the beginning, not to run. If your running partner is unable to run, or has to postpone a run, you are likely to give it a miss. It is best to run with someone who has a little experience and who is a little faster than you to keep you on your toes and push you to your limit. But do not run with someone who is much faster, it is too discouraging.

It is better for a woman to run with another woman, as running can cause family discord when a woman tries to keep up with her husband and strains herself. She may feel she is holding him back. He may try to run too slowly and get frustrated, or feel guilty if he goes too far ahead. It is better for a faster runner to go on ahead and then double back from time to time to pick the other up.

Running Muggers

Some women are very worried about being mugged while out jogging alone. Most muggers prefer beating up frail old ladies. They know runners do not carry money or handbags and that a lady runner is also strong enough to stand her own ground or fast enough to escape. First, a would-be mugger has to catch his prey and there are not too many criminal runners about.

If you are nervous of running alone, run in built-up areas. Tell someone your route and what time you plan to return.

What to Wear

Your running kit is important. You need a good pair of running shoes with a 'gristle' rubber sole and soft leather or nylon upper, and a wedge of firm rubber to pad the heels. The heavier you are the more you need to cushion the heel to absorb the jolt of each step. Shoes should fit firmly but not tightly, and allow at least an extra half inch in the toes. Nike Equator and Nike Transit are very good shoes.

The right kind of socks are also important. Socks with seams may cause blisters so may socks which are too thin or too small. Splash out on Nike cotton socks which are soft and absorbent.

You can always start with an old pair of tennis plimsols. I started in ordinary walking shoes.

A smart tracksuit or running shorts and T-shirt are useful. Again I use Nike which has the natural fibres to absorb the sweat. Have it loose fitting to allow air to circulate to help keep you cool, and make sure nothing chafes. After 10 or 15 miles a rough edge to a sleeve can cause a painful sore. Most of all it is important that you look good because it will help you feel good and give you the right attitude to your running and your life.

Taking the first step is obviously crucial. There are always reasons for not going out when you are under pressure. This is the time, of course, when you need to go out most of all.

Bruce Tulloh, the Olympics coach, uses a few mutters to put him in the right frame of mind. 'Five o'clock is running time.' 'Running makes the heart grow stronger. Running is fun, running is life.' I used to say, 'Running is hope, running is to survive.'

When you are fit you will run effortlessly and feel you are flying. You may not do very well at first, you may want to turn round and go home, but you have done better than the person who is still thinking about it.

Goals

My stepson Michael was nursing a New Year's Day hangover. I asked him if he had any New Year's resolutions. 'Yes,' he said. 'My goal in life is to feel better.'

Everyone needs a goal and to feel better. Like Michael you need a specific target so you can judge your progress. This should be governed by your state of fitness. You may decide you want to run 2 miles in twenty minutes, or just make it to the end of your road. My ultimate goal was the Marathon, but before that I entered for Fun Runs. The first was 3 miles, then 5 miles and so on.

Time each run or walk over a measured distance and record your progress in a diary. In my diary I used little codes: NB – no booze; NB & F – no booze and fags; W – withdrawal symptoms, i.e. a hangover; A – aggravation, i.e., a row with my husband.

Record everything at the beginning, then you will find out what suits you or what holds you back. Keeping to a set programme is an achievement in itself. You have still done better than the person who has done nothing at all or gave up halfway.

The difference between jogging and running is speed. A fast walk is 4 miles an hour, a slow jog is 5 or 6 miles an hour or ten to twelve minutes per mile. Most people feel comfortable jogging around 6 or 7 miles an hour. Running is 8 to 10 miles an hour.

Jogging has fashions and trends like everything else; at the moment most people prefer to talk of running rather than jogging.

Pre-Run Exercise

Before you run do stretching exercises to warm up. The first ten minutes of any run is the hardest. It can be made a little easier with limbering-up exercises. But, however hard the first minutes, you must remember that it always gets better. Your body has to get used to the demands you are asking of it. During a five-minute run, the first two minutes are hell; during a marathon it is the first 3 miles.

The end of a run can also be hard going, particularly if you are pushing yourself to the limit. When I ran the Marathon I found the first 2 miles difficult and the last 2 miles almost impossible – but I still enjoyed the total experience.

After the Run

What happens directly after your run is important. Do not spoil your relaxed good mood, give yourself time to bathe and change before embarking on pressurized activity. You will be able to cope much better.

Walk around after you have stopped rushing to avoid cooling down too quickly. I usually make myself a large cup of coffee (you may prefer a cold drink, orange juice or milk) while my bath is running. I take the coffee and the tape cassette into the bathroom, ritually pour in the bath oil and enjoy a leisurely soak, one that I've earned. I drink my coffee and listen to music. I then get dressed slowly and start the day.

As you progress and tackle longer runs, 10 or 13 miles, you may find that you are pushing your body quite hard for the first time. There can be some worrying after-effects. Watch for the signs of dehydration and hypothermia. This is lack of water and body heat. You can lose body heat very rapidly and your brain tends to go numb.

If I plan to have a hard run, I make sure I have a blanket or fresh tracksuit to put on as soon as I get in.

I have a special high-protein drink ready in the refrigerator and I keep moving until I can get into a hot bath. To get a fast return of energy I prepare a special drink I call a Life Reviver, recommended by my coach Tony.

Life Reviver
For 2 people:
6 dessertspoons of Sportive Protein Power powder
1 pint skimmed milk
3 eggs
1 dessertspoonful of honey
1 banana

Place the ingredients in the blender and liquidize. Pour into two glasses and chill. This can be varied with half milk and half ice cream. I found a delicious variation was to use tinned guavas instead of banana, but any fruit will do.

You can buy the Sportive products or the equivalent from gyms and body-building centres, some health-food shops and sports centres.

Starting to Run

Before you run, measure a route in your car, starting and finishing if possible at your front door. The route should be at least a mile long and ideally include grass verges and a moderate hill.

Most of us, including myself at 20 stone, can walk a mile. When my stepson Randal wrote his first week's training instructions, he did not want anything to seem too difficult to put me off. He didn't want me to do anything of which I was not capable. You should start small but then build up.

My first week's instructions for running a marathon were encouragingly simple:

Sunday	Go for a walk. Time it and report.
Monday	Walk five minutes briskly.
Tuesday	Walk five minutes slowly.
Wednesday	Walk ten minutes slowly.
Thursday	Walk fifteen minutes (stop and rest if you want).
Friday	Rest
Saturday	Walk five minutes.

Drink as much as you like but do not exceed more than one bottle of vodka a day; drink as much wine as you like. Eat as much as you like.

I carried out these instructions. I continued to walk for two months until my weight was down to about 17½ stone. My walks got longer each week. I was careful to walk four mornings a week for at least fifteen minutes and then have a long walk at the weekend, between 2 and 7 miles.

To become fit and healthy it is not necessary to run a marathon. To become fit and lose weight and maintain your weight loss, however, you will need to be able to run at least 5 miles in fifty minutes. This is enough to turn an unfit person into a 'runner'. It is also the foundation for greater things.

If you want to run a marathon after you have made the 5-mile mark, training should take place over a period of three months gradually building up to a minimum of 50 miles a week with one long run a week of up to 22 miles.

My training was based on the schedule in Bruce Tulloh's *The Complete Jogger*. Randal and I adapted the regime to suit my needs and this I pass on to you.

I am going to assume you can walk for 1 mile. Set a weekly objective, the first week to cover 1 mile in thirty minutes.

Week One

Monday	Walk slowly round the mile circuit and time yourself.
Tuesday	Walk at normal pace round the mile circuit and time yourself.
Wednesday	Rest.
Thursday	Alternately walk slowly and briskly round the circuit. Five minutes fast, five minutes slow.
Friday	Walk briskly round the circuit.
Saturday	Walk briskly for half a mile, jog slowly for thirty seconds. Walk until you recover your normal breathing rate, then jog again for

	thirty seconds. Walk home slowly. Time
	yourself. Compare your time on Saturday
	with your Monday time.
Sunday	Rest.

Geoffrey Cannon, the writer of *New Health* and Director of the Great British Fun Run, told me he believed some runners benefit from running every other day, particularly beginners and those over thirty-five years of age. I agree with Geoffrey that it is not necessarily the amount of running you do, but the quality. I am sure, for example, that older runners can benefit from a day of rest between runs. I know, however, that when I started I needed to run nearly every day.

If I missed one day, I was liable to miss another and another. Until you really get going, it is best to restrict rest days to once or twice a week and never allow more than one day to lapse between runs.

You should be able to complete your first week without strain. If you are particularly breathless during jogging, see your doctor. If you do not complete any of the week's training, repeat that week.

Randal kept telling me to 'train, don't strain'. Above all, keep to the schedule, but do not overdo things at the beginning.

Week Two
The objective is to cover 1 mile in twenty minutes.

Monday	Establish a pattern of walking and jogging
	round your mile circuit: 300 yards at brisk
	walk, 100 yards jog, 50 yards walk. Repeat
	three times.
Tuesday	Repeat Monday but try to increase your
	jogging distance to about 150 yards. I used to
	fix on a gatepost or tree as my finishing line

	for the jog. Each day I tried to go just a little bit further, only a few steps, but it is better to go further than faster.
Wednesday	Increase the distance you are covering to 1½ miles. You could just go on for an extra five minutes, and back again, which should be about an extra half mile. Try more walking than jogging on this run.
Thursday	Rest.
Friday	A 2-mile walk. Do not attempt to jog and try to take about fifty minutes. Walk round your mile circuit twice, although it is a good idea to have several different routes worked out of different duration.
Saturday	Testing day. A brisk walk to cover the mile in twenty minutes without breaking into a jog. If you can do faster, so much the better, but do not try to over-extend yourself. An injury can set you back for weeks and is never worth it.
Sunday	Rest.

You should be comfortable walking 2 miles. You should now be wearing good running shoes and socks and a loose-fitting tracksuit. If any of your joints ache, rest for a couple of days and start Week Two again.

Week Three
Stepping up the mileage is the way to improve speed and stamina. The aim is to cover 6 miles during the week and a mile in eighteen minutes.

| Monday | Cover 1½ miles. Jog for thirty seconds. Increase the number of thirty-second jogs to |

	four in the 1½ miles.
Tuesday	1½ miles. This time increase your distance each time. Jog for 150 yards or fifty seconds four times. You should be able to recover with a brisk walk rather than a slow one.
Wednesday	2 miles. Stride out for a mile. Do not use too much energy too early. Jog for two thirty-second bursts. Walk the last half mile home.
Thursday	Rest.
Friday	1½ miles again. Jog a longer distance – anything from 110 yards to 150 yards. Walk slowly for 50 yards and briskly until your breathing is quite normal. Repeat six times.
Saturday	Test yourself again. Cover 1 mile in eighteen minutes. Repeat the previous day's formula and remember to write your distance and times in your diary to compare with the beginning of the week.
Sunday	Rest.

If you have reached your target and feel nothing more than slight discomfort, you are doing well. If in doubt, or you did not complete the training, repeat the week.

You may find that your legs are fine but your breathing difficult, or the other way round. Cut down on cigarettes or try to give them up for a while. Concentrate on slow regular breaths. Do not be worried by the sound. Breathe in and blow out slowly and regularly, and pace your running to suit your breathing. You can strengthen your legs with leg exercises or aerobics, and weight training.

Week Four
The objective is to cover 1 mile in fifteen minutes.

Monday	A long walk, 3 miles. Walk briskly and run on a flat surface. You could go three times round your 1-mile circuit, or try a new route. It is good to vary your route runs, to experience different terrain. It is tempting to pick a flat route, but hills should be included although it is unwise to try running up hills at this stage.
Tuesday	1½ miles running and walking, with 150-yard jogs (fifty seconds), repeated six times.
Wednesday	2 miles walking and jogging. 150-yard jog repeated six times.
Thursday	Rest.
Friday	1½ miles walking and jogging. Extend your jogging time a few steps with each spurt. Cut down on the slow walking time and walk briskly for most of the run.
Saturday	Cover 1 mile in fifteen minutes. Notice how much shorter the mile has become? So much easier than when you first started.
Sunday	Rest.

The purpose of this training schedule is to get you into shape, fit enough to feel good, lose weight and to continue with more strenuous running. The aim is a ten-minute mile over a 5-mile distance. Because of the weight I was carrying, I found I was progressing well in covering the miles but always taking longer than I expected. The only way for me to speed up was to lose weight.

To progress you must follow my diet to lose weight. The lighter you become the faster you run with the minimum of effort. The faster you run, the quicker you lose weight.

A fat person has to make a greater effort to cover the same distance than a thin person. This is tiresome but a terrific bonus in the long run. When slim, everything is so much easier and you have all that extra effort in your 'running bank'; this means your tolerance over the long runs would be greater than that of a slim person.

Do not worry if you are not making the time trials; as long as you are improving and covering the distance you do not need to repeat a week as before.

Week Five
Two miles in thirty minutes is the aim. The magical ten-minute mile will soon be in sight. This week will be quite a bit harder than previous weeks.

Monday	Walk 3 miles briskly in forty-five minutes. Try doing it in your lunch hour instead of lunch. When you are training you are not eating.
Tuesday	1½ miles of walking and jogging. Aim to step up the distance you are jogging.
Wednesday	2 miles walking and jogging. You should now be doing 50 per cent jogging to brisk walking. You should try to cut out the slow walking altogether. Do not try to run again until you have recovered from your previous run.
Thursday	Rest.
Friday	1½ miles running and walking.
Saturday	Time trial over 2 miles. Twice round a 1-mile circuit. You are better able to judge your speed on a familiar route. You should be running two fifteen-minute miles. Write down your time in your diary and compare with your time five weeks ago. You will be pleasantly surprised.
Sunday	Rest.

You should be able to manage this running programme on either the 1-pound-a-week diet or the 3-pound-a-week diet. I find it better not to eat before running, but then I usually run in the morning. You should not eat less than two hours before, however. Apart from the discomfort there is the very real likelihood of being sick, particularly if you are pushing yourself.

After a very hard run you can still feel very sick even on an empty stomach. If you do feel sick afterwards, you are probably going too hard.

Week Six
Four miles in a hour is the aim.

Monday	Walk 4 miles briskly. Try going cross-country for a bit, it is easier on the legs, although it may be harder and take longer initially. Running along grass verges also saves wear and tear on knees and ankles.
Tuesday	1 mile walking and running. Walk 200 yards, run 200 yards, walk 50 yards slowly and 150 yards briskly. You should do at least four 200-yard runs per mile.
Wednesday	2 miles walking and running, the same pattern as Tuesday. Try to increase your running distance each time. This strengthens the heart and lung muscles.
Thursday	Rest. Some people prefer to have just one day off a week.
	If you want to train on a rest day I suggest a gentle half-mile run. It is important, though, that you have at least one whole day off a week. A rest day should be just that. Do not think that because you are not running, you can play squash instead. If you want to

play an additional sport do it on a day when your training is fairly light. By now you may begin to feel, as I do, that a day has not really started without a run, however brief.

Friday	1 mile walking and running.
Saturday	Time trial. 4 miles in one hour.
Sunday	Rest; this means no hard physical activities.

We all develop at different rates. You may start slowly as I did, but then progress quickly as you get fitter. If in doubt, repeat a week's training schedule. I repeated this week's schedule twice. Some weeks I repeated three times.

Week Seven
Five miles in one hour is the aim.

Monday	Walk 5 miles briskly, try a little running.
Tuesday	Run and walk 1 mile. 200 yards jog, 200 yards walk. Take it easy.
Wednesday	2 miles walking and running. Step up your speed a little.
Thursday	Rest.
Friday	1 mile running. Take it easy.
Saturday	Time trial. Walk and run 5 miles in under one hour. You will probably find that you are now running almost all the distance. In future long runs should take place at the weekend or when you have the extra time.
Sunday	Rest.

Week Eight
The aim this week is to run 1 mile in ten minutes. The ten-minute mile is the standard on which all future running is based. When you can run a mile in ten minutes, you have already

reached an acceptable state of fitness.

Monday	Walk 5 miles briskly.
Tuesday	Run and walk 1 mile. You should now be running most of the way. If not, run 250 yards, walk 200 yards.
Wednesday	Run and walk 2 miles. Remember to keep running very slowly. If you have trouble in raising the distance you are running, try to slow down your pace. One of the hardest things to do is run slowly and pace yourself.
Thursday	Rest.
Friday	2 mile running and walking. Try going a bit faster.
Saturday	Your time trial. You must jog non-stop for 1 mile in ten minutes.
Sunday	Rest.

If you succeed with this week's training, you have come to the end of the beginning. With all milestones, though, you must ensure that you can maintain and sustain this speed. Over the next three or four weeks you must build up your speed over the distance.

Week Nine
Your aim is to run 3 miles in 30 minutes.

Monday	Walk and run 6 miles.
Tuesday	Run only 1 mile.
Wednesday	Walk and run 3 miles.
Thursday	Rest.
Friday	Walk and run 2 miles.
Saturday	Your time trial. Walk and run 3 miles in thirty minutes. You should be running nearly all the way.
Sunday	Rest.

You may find at this stage, as I did, that you have made a breakthrough with your training. There may also be weeks when nothing seems to happen. Do not be discouraged, if you have hit a sticky patch, you may be over-tired. Take a couple of days off and try again.

Week Ten
Five miles in 50 minutes is the aim.

Monday	Walk and run 6 miles.
Tuesday	Run 1 mile slowly.
Wednesday	Walk and run 3 miles.
Thursday	Rest.
Friday	Walk and run 2 miles.
Saturday	Walk and run 5 miles in 50 minutes.
Sunday	Rest.

Congratulations. Training has stepped up. You should now be fitter and slimmer and able to cope with a lot more. If you are still more than 20 pounds overweight, you may be doing slower times but, nevertheless, you are still capable of keeping to the schedule and doing better times.

Danger Signs

It is not always easy to tell if you are pushing yourself too hard. Tiredness is accumulative so it is necessary to know the symptoms of a build-up to exhaustion. Tiredness may be your problem. Here are some indicators.
1. Reduced performance, you are getting slower and not faster; you have a raised heart rate.
2. Sore muscles, particularly in the thighs.
3. Increased tendency to infection, colds, etc.

4. Increased irritability.
5. Lack of concentration and difficulty in sitting still for any length of time.
6. Stomach disorders, either diarrhoea or constipation.
7. Loss of appetite (rare in my case).
8. Accelerated weight loss.
9. Difficulty in co-ordinating movements while running.
10. Lack of a desire to train, and difficulty in sleeping, general lethargy.

If you experience several of these symptoms together, reduce your training load.

If you experience an abnormal heart action while running, an irregular pulse, fluttering, pumping or palpitations of the throat or chest, stop exercising and see your doctor at once.

If you feel faint during exercise, sit down immediately and put your head between your knees and then see your doctor. Also if you suffer pain or pressure in the chest, arm or throat, stop exercising and again consult your doctor.

Most of the symptoms can usually be treated with a rest from training for two or three days. When you return to your programme, start again at the beginning of the week and take it very easily.

If a complete rest is needed, perhaps with a leg injury, you could try swimming as an alternative. This is less strenuous and will not aggravate muscle strain; it will also prevent you slipping back with your training. Once you have really got started with a few miles 'in the bank', a few days off do not seriously erode your fitness. Getting going again may seem a little hard at first, but you will be back to your old standard after a couple of good runs. Unless you have to stop training for several weeks, you do not lose your fitness easily.

Injuries

I have been remarkably free of injuries since I started to run. Indeed, injuries are the exception rather than the rule.

Most of the aches and twinges you experience are your body adjusting itself. I did have a problem when I was very overweight with my knees, particularly down steep hills. This was cured by resting for seven days and then running on level grass rather than roads for a couple of weeks.

Other ailments, strained tendons and pulled muscles have usually been incurred through some different activity. The fitter you get the more you attempt. I pulled my Achilles tendon on one occasion doing stretching exercises. Another time I pulled a muscle by dancing too enthusiastically. It is important you take all exercises gently, especially squash. All movement should be gradual and smooth so as not to jolt your body.

Blisters: these are often caused by the wrong type of socks rather than by poor shoes, and can afflict all parts of the body besides the feet. I used to get bad blisters round my bra straps and where my sleeve rubbed. Different clothing and vaseline should help.

Neck and shoulder strain: this is due to over-rigidity when running and can be prevented with gentle loosening-up exercises, rotating the head and swinging the arms. Try to lower your shoulders and run in a relaxed way.

Wrenched ankles: these may be caused by running on uneven surfaces and should be rested completely until better.

Cramps: these are probably the most common running ailment and can be disastrous in a big run. Leg cramps usually occur after a run and can be avoided by cooling down slowly, keeping on the move and keeping warm. Stomach cramps are a different problem and are often a sign that you are running too fast or are exhausted. Usually I slow down, grit my teeth and run through a cramp; sometimes it works but not always.

Occasionally you may just have to walk or even drop out of a race.

Weight Training

I found it invaluable to visit a gymnasium three times a week while I was training. It improved my stamina, helped my breathing and firmed up my body, so that the 'slack' from the weight loss was kept to a minimum. The gymnasium was also a refuge from the temptations of eating.

Many people may find difficulty in finding time to go to a gym, but a couple of visits should give you a training programme that you could do at home.

I was very fortunate when I went to the Olympian Studio in Bournemouth. Tony, the manager who became my trainer, gave me exercises to do, tailored to my needs, for both the gym and my home. Most good gyms will do this and it is worthwhile investing in a couple of 10-kilo hand-weights to have at home.

Weight training does not build up unsightly muscle; the secret is to get to a basic level with the weights, then not increase the weight, but only the number of times you repeat the exercise. That way you get fitness, firmness and stamina without looking like Charles Atlas.

After a good work-out, you can usually reward yourself with a sauna and a massage. I used to have these at both the Olympian, in Bournemouth, and the Roman Rooms in Ringwood where I discovered the delights of a friendly mixed sauna. Massages are a wonderful luxury. There is nothing that your poor tired muscles will appreciate more.

Holidays

Respect local customs and the heat. Too much sun or humidity is dangerous. Be careful not to raise your body temperature too much. Do not lie in the sun before running, be sure to be cool before you start, and replace the water you have lost as soon as you stop.

In many countries, particularly the Arab states, it will cause trouble if a woman runs in shorts and T-shirt. It is anyway better to run in Arab-style clothing, light-coloured djellabas or baggy trousers to protect you from the heat and reflect the rays of the sun. You may need those potassium pills now to replace the salt and minerals lost while sweating.

To run in a cold country, wrap up well, perhaps two tracksuits (one hooded) plus shorts and T-shirt and shoes which are big enough to take extra-thick socks which should not cramp the feet. Clothes should be loose fitting. I now have an excellent Gor-Tex running suit which protects me from the rain but allows the body to breathe and keeps me very warm. The prices are high but will soon be coming down.

Fun Runs

At a certain point in your training you will feel ready to compete. This is why they invented fun runs. We are like children who want to show the grown-ups how well we've done.

The Fun Run also acts as confirmation of a standard of running you have achieved.

The first Fun Run can be rather nerve-racking, but worth it for the pride of achievement you feel afterwards.

Pick a 3- or 5-mile Fun Run as a goal for when you have completed your programme. Your first Fun Run should be a big affair, preferably with children so that you can be sure to come ahead of somebody and be able to get lost in the crowd. At the beginning I think it is important not to come last but, later on, I happily trundled in after the last runner in a top-class road race, knowing that my competition was tough.

Select a run near you, from *Running* magazine or your local newspaper or sports centre.

Stoking Up

For the Fun Runner I recommend that two or three days before a race you start to eat more carbohydrates, preferably pasta, bread and potatoes, but the odd biscuit or pudding would be excusable. Be careful not to gain more than 4 ounces for each mile you are running or you might not lose the weight you've gained so easily.

On a Fun Run you may find water stations *en route* for the first time. Do be sure you do not drink too much before a race as you could be running off to the nearest loo during the race. You probably do not need to take on water during a run for anything less than 13 miles but, on the whole, you will feel better if you drink while running, particularly in the early stages of the race. Do not drink more than a pint an hour before the race.

Be sure to wear clothes and shoes which are already broken in, or you could end up with blisters. Vaseline anything that might chafe: between the thighs, bra straps, feet, and under the arms.

On a Fun Run you may find water stations *en route* for the first home afterwards. You will always run faster in competitive running and may well push yourself pretty hard. You need someone waiting at the finish with a tracksuit and a drink. Although most runs nowadays provide good water and baggage facilities, there is no substitute for a friend to scoop you up, prop you up, tell you how well you did, and take you home. It is no fun driving a long distance after a very hard run.

Hash House Harriers

Running introduces you to a lot of new people.

There is the weekend executive runner who is trying to offset all those weekday expense-account lunches. Some runners quite like the idea of escaping from their spouses for a while. There are those who are looking for new friends or partners and see running as a social club where a strained hamstring or hitting the wall is a qualification for membership.

Then there are the backsliders who want to get rid of the chocolate cake and beer and the hangover from the night before. There are also the serious runners who talk about running all the time and know about every race that was ever run.

Recently I joined an organization which has all these types, the Wessex Hash House Harriers. The Wessex Hash is a chapter of an international organization for runners who do it purely for fun. We meet every Sunday, often in a pub deep in the heart of the New Forest.

We then spend a couple of hours running across fields and through woods and streams following a trail of sawdust previously laid by two hashers called 'hares'. It is always wet and muddy with a long run of about 7 miles and a shorter one, for less experienced runners, of 3 miles. The run terminates at the pub, the hashers then take off all their muddy clothes in their cars, dress as ordinary human beings and swarm into the pub to undo all the good the two-hour run has done. Various obscure rituals then take place. The hares and other unfortunates are forced to drink large quantities of beer or lemonade from a mug or chamber pot at the instigation of the Grand Master and encouraged with ribald singing from the rest of the gathering.

The Hash House Harriers claim to be a responsible body of men and women dedicated to flattening fields and disrupting Sunday Services. They are also wonderful company and very good fun. Food and drink, tasted after a hard hash, is most delicious. A 7-mile cross-country run works up an appetite that turns the humble ploughman's lunch into *haute cuisine*. The relaxed silliness afterwards is exactly right to smooth away the tensions of the week. With the Wessex Hash I have seen the most beautiful countryside in Britain. It is altogether a rewarding, harmless and rather eccentric pastime with some amiable and harmless eccentrics.

Does It Improve Your Sex Life?

Apart from the actual sexual stimulus of running – the 'runner's high' – there is a vast improvement in most runners' sex lives.

The exercise does strengthen your cardio-vascular system which pumps blood to the heart, lungs and all parts of the body; this makes everything much more efficient. There is truth in the T-shirt slogan: 'Marathon runners keep it up for hours.' My husband confirms you do not need to run a marathon, just 3 miles three times a week is quite good enough.

With my new body and added zest I feel much more desirable. We are both livelier, more relaxed and vital but, above all, more aware of each other.